D1189493

STRESS AND DISEASE

HAROLD G. WOLFF'S
STRESS AND DISEASE

Second Edition

Revised and Edited by

STEWART WOLF, M.D.

Regents Professor of Medicine and Psychiatry
University of Oklahoma Medical Center
Oklahoma City, Oklahoma

and

HELEN GOODELL, B.S.

Research Associate, Department of Neurology
Cornell-New York Hospital Medical Center
New York, New York

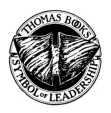

CHARLES C THOMAS • PUBLISHER
Springfield • Illinois • U.S.A.

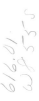

Published and Distributed Throughout the World by

CHARLES C THOMAS • PUBLISHER

BANNERSTONE HOUSE

301-327 East Lawrence Avenue, Springfield, Illinois, U.S.A.

NATCHEZ PLANTATION HOUSE

735 North Atlantic Boulevard, Fort Lauderdale, Florida, U.S.A.

This book is protected by copyright. No part of it may be reproduced in any manner without written permission from the publisher.

© *1953 and 1968, by* CHARLES C THOMAS • PUBLISHER

Library of Congress Catalog Card Number: 66-21439

First Edition, 1953

Second Edition, 1968

With **THOMAS BOOKS** *careful attention is given to all details of manufacturing and design. It is the Publisher's desire to present books that are satisfactory as to their physical qualities and artistic possibilities and appropriate for their particular use.* **THOMAS BOOKS** *will be true to those laws of quality that assure a good name and good will.*

Printed in the United States of America

G-2

DEDICATION

To
ISABEL BISHOP WOLFF
*whose lively sensitive mind, creativity,
encouragement, criticism and
deep devotion contributed richly
to her husband's great work*

INTRODUCTION

THE FIRST EDITION of Harold G. Wolff's *Stress and Disease* was published in 1952. By 1960 the book was already out of print, and new data in the rapidly developing field required that a new edition be prepared. Dr. Wolff agreed to write a second edition, planning to revise completely the old format. He had in mind a scientific essay that would be intelligible to the educated layman as well as to the scientist and practitioner. He envisioned not only a general description of experimental studies but a major emphasis on interpretation and on the development of the concept of the ecology of man. At the time of his death in 1962, he had gathered much material. In the meantime, also, he had delivered three major lectures on which he planned to draw heavily for the text of the book. The organization of the book had not gone far enough, however, to make it possible for a substitute author to develop Dr. Wolff's plan without doing violence to it. Therefore, when Charles C Thomas, Publisher and Mrs. Harold G. Wolff, requested that I prepare the second edition of *Stress and Disease,* it seemed wisest to stick to the original concept, presenting the experimental data but broadening somewhat the interpretation and including considerable material from the three lectures. I asked Helen Goodell, the person who had shared most closely Harold Wolff's scientific adventures over the years and who best understood his thinking, to collaborate in the preparation of this second edition. For both of us, it has been a labor of love and an opportunity to pay tribute to our chief, an outstanding experimental scientist and intellectual leader.

We have enlarged the scope of the first edition to include a systematic presentation of protective, adaptive reactions in all of the body systems that have been brought under study by Harold Wolff or his former pupils now widely distributed over the United States, and as far afield as Canada, Europe, and the

Middle East, Japan, India, and Australia. We also decided to prepare a detailed presentation of methodology since it was the approach and the creative way of attacking important questions that as much as anything else distinguished Harold Wolff's investigations. "Fixity of purpose requires flexibility of method" was his motto. In Chapter II, we have attempted to describe the extraordinary range and resourcefulness of his methods and those of his students. Finally, we have attempted to bring the book together with a consideration of the mechanisms of the brain as they relate to the regulation and control of the organs and the systems of the body, and thereby to bodily disturbances and disease.

Doctor Wolff died at the Clinical Center of the National Institutes of Health at Bethesda, Maryland, in February, 1962, of a massive cerebral thrombosis. He was attending a meeting on cerebrovascular disease. It is ironic that his first scientific studies conducted at Harvard with H. S. Forbes and Stanley Cobb had concerned the cranial vasculature. His focus of interest on the cranial vessels persisted and culminated in his classical studies of migraine and of the mechanisms of headache. The second edition of his monumental treatise on headache had been just about completed at the time of his death.

Although sixty-three years old when he died, Harold Wolff's creative life was in full flower. While most men hit their stride somewhere along in middle-life, maintain a plateau for a time, adding little to their accomplishments and ultimately decline, Wolff was on a steep portion of his own intellectual growth curve at the time of his death. His interests had broadened and deepened at the same time, and his capacity for understanding man and his condition was growing apace. Still rapidly learning, he incorporated into his scheme of thought whatever he could use to build a clearer understanding of human ecology as it relates to health and disease. His prehensile mind would pick out significant items in all manner of literature—scientific, historical, or documentary and from conversations with all manner of observant men—scholars, scientists, sportsmen, and explorers. Thus, with his stupendous grasp of ideas and his incorruptible respect for evidence Harold Wolff succeeded in molding an original concept of disease that influenced the thinking and the growth of many productive people who were close to him and indeed the pattern of thought of a whole generation of medicine. The full impact of Harold Wolff's contributions will be increasingly felt as the years pass. Meanwhile, it is our hope that this volume will do justice to him and to his work. It is offered with affection and deep respect for his memory.

The authors are grateful to Oxford University Press, the Williams and Wilkins Company, Paul B. Hoeber, Charles C Thomas, Publisher, The Association for Research in Nervous and Mental Disease, *Transactions of the Association of American Physicians, Journal of Clinical Investigation, American Journal of the Medical Sciences, The Archives of Neurology and Psychiatry, Neurology, The Journal of Laboratory and Clinical Medicine,* and *The Transactions of the American Clinical and Climatological Association* for permission to reproduce figures and text material.

Special thanks are due Mary Steichen and Virgene Ficken for their careful secretarial work at every stage in the development of the manuscript, and to Harriet Ross, who checked and corrected the galleys.

S. W.
H. G.

CONTENTS

STRESS AND DISEASE

Chapter I

THE NATURE OF STRESS FOR MAN

HAZARDS IN HIS ENVIRONMENT

MAN IS EXPOSED to assaults by other living forms that aim to invade as parasites or to destroy; by meteorological and climatic crises that pass sometimes predictably and often with seeming whimsey over the earth's surface; by other physical forces that affect man merely in terms of his mass and volume; and by elements of the earth's crust which man often dangerously manipulates for his sustenance and fulfillment, comfort and delight, or to vent his passion for dominion (1-4).

Man is vulnerable because he reacts not only to the actual existence of danger, but to threats and symbols of danger experienced in his past. Pavlov, while studying the secretory function of the stomach in dogs, suddenly found his observations of responses to standard stimuli completely distorted following a violent thunderstorm that flooded the kennels (5, 6). He was then obliged to infer that activities of the stomach are so dependent upon the animal's reactions to conditions in the kennels and laboratories before and during observation, that understanding of digestive secretion requires an evaluation of the significance of these "conditions" to the animal.

Sometimes, threats evoke reactions of long duration and even of greater magnitude than the assault itself. The resulting protective adaptive reaction, when sustained, may be far more damaging to the individual than the effects of the noxious agent per se. The adaptive capabilities of any individual are necessarily limited in kind. A man's response to many sorts of noxious agents and threats may be similar, the form of the reaction to any one agent depending more on the individual's nature, past experience and future goals than upon the particular noxious agent evoking

it. Nineteenth century descriptive pathologists carried out histologic analysis to the point where it seemed possible that in the
not too far distant future, with further advance in microscopy,
every tissue alteration could be linked with a specific etiological
agent. The subsequent development of the electron microscope
has not justified this hope. Moreover, during the twentieth century, with the growth of experimental pathology, thought has
continued to move quite sharply in the opposite direction to an
awareness that grossly different agents may evoke indistinguishable reactions in the host (7) ; and that reactions of great magnitude may result from situations that are ordinarily benign,
because of the peculiar significance of the stimuli to the individual involved (8).

A CONCEPT OF STRESS

Although long used in common language with a variety of
meaning, the word "stress" has been given by physicists a precise
definition as it applies to the mechanics of non-living systems,
i.e., stress is the cohesive force or molecular resistance in a body
opposing the action of applied external force (9). The resem-
blance to the situation in living systems is remote. Yet, figuratively the concept is useful, and when employed in reference to
human problems merely implies an analogy to the order in non-
living systems. Since stress is a dynamic state within an organism
in response to a demand for adaptation, and since life itself entails
constant adaptations, living creatures are continually in a state
of more or less stress. The objective of this volume is to examine
the nature of adaptive responses, the consequences thereof, and
their modifiability.

With an awareness of the importance of the direct effects of
climate, micro-organisms, terrain, chemical and physical forces
in disease, emphasis in this essay will be placed upon those
alterations within the human host that stem from exposure to
changes and challenges of many varieties; from disruption of
customs and habits as well as familial and social structures; from
the deprivation of basic human needs (interpersonal and esthetic)
and the failure to give expression to human proclivities. Also,

focus will be upon the alterations in the vulnerability of tissue resulting from threats to life, threats of deprivation of the basic needs and of opportunities for growth, development and fulfillment of human potentialities (10-14).

The changes, disruptions, deprivations, hindrances and threats result mainly from the interaction of men with one another, both singly and in groups (15-21). Moreover, the adaptive responses so evoked may be indistinguishable from those induced by more tangible forces and, indeed, responses may combine with additive effect (22-24).

Although stress is commonly thought of as destructive, it is not necessarily so (25-27). Frustration and misfortune may lead, and perhaps be essential to the growth and strengthening of a person, just as they may also lead to maladaptive reactions (28).

In studying patterns of reaction that may have pathogenic significance, it is customary to think of struggle, excessive effort, striving, catastrophe, drama and violence, revolution and upheavals as accompanied by feelings of anxiety, panic and despair. Actually, though such events and reactions are relevant to our discussions, others equally relevant may appear ostensibly so mundane and the accompanying reactions so devoid of evident feeling content, that many individuals may deny the presence or significance of both. Yet, those very same subjects may be reacting to their life circumstances in a manner that leads to illness. More than surface inspection is often necessary to identify the meaning to an individual of seemingly benign circumstances, events or demands. Especially significant to this recognition is the factor of timing, i.e., the time of life in relation to other events, the rate of occurrence, the phase of environmental social change or individual social mobility, the historic moment and the resulting significance of familial, social and cultural demands. With consideration of the facets of man's nature, his habits and his way of life, a better understanding of his diseases becomes possible (29-34).

THE NATURE OF STIMULI AND REACTIONS

The word "noxious," when related to stimulus, implies that

its effects may be harmful not only as regards integrity of tissues but even with respect to individual health or survival (25). Among noxious stimuli may be included a variety of threats and symbols of danger, as well as clear demands for a change in the pattern of intimate relationships, such as the first love affair, marriage, birth of a child, retirement, a change of job, a promotion, and such calamitous events as death of a loved one, loss of a job, or the outbreak of war. Such stressful situations may jeopardize health or even survival.

Stimuli in the category of symbols can be defined as noxious only if they are so perceived by the individual implicated. One cannot apply the term "noxious" to a situation merely on the basis of the physical, interpersonal and social alterations in the environment of the individual. The situation takes on noxious significance only in terms of its meaning to the individual based on his innate characteristics, his past experience and future goals. This limited use of the word "noxious," then, aims to avoid the confusion that follows when one is confronted with the fact that illness may prove to be an asset in one way or another. For example, the illnesses of Charles Darwin and of Florence Nightingale may have been motivating factors in their respective creative efforts that produced the *Origin of Species* and reforms in hospital nursing. Other individuals, while perceiving the noxious nature of their experiences may nevertheless respond with utter disregard, as if they could glimpse some ultimate good to society for which they are driven to pay the price of broken health or even loss of life. Though it is necessary to connect "noxious" with individual experience, nevertheless, most of us in a given culture perceive in common many symbols as dangerous and react to them in one way or another that may lead to illness. There may even be, at some given time in history or in a particular cultural group, a prevailing type of reaction involving illness, as for example, peptic ulceration or tuberculosis (See Chapt. VI, p. 191). In short, the word "noxious" is useful because it allows one to deal with two broad varieties of stimuli; direct or unconditioned, and indirect or conditioned. This permits a continuum in a formulation that would otherwise contain an awkward dichotomy, and gives a clue as to which of all sorts of circumstances can be seen to be relevant to disease. In this frame of reference it also becomes clear why "one man's meat is another man's poison," and allows a view of human reaction patterns which would include those of the "commando" who has been so trained to court danger and violence that an horrendous situation produces relatively little untoward effect; and those of the paranoid individual who may perceive a life endangering threat in a bystander's innocent allusion.

Central to the problem of stress for man, with his elaborate use of symbols, is his special sensitivity about his place in the eyes of other men. Man is a tribal creature with a long period of development, and depends for his very existence on the aid, support and the real and symbolic encouragement of other men. He lives his life so much in contact with others and he is so deeply concerned about their expectations of him, that perhaps his greatest threat is their disapproval and rejection.

Man is threatened by those very forces in society upon which he is dependent for nourishment and life. He must be part of the tribe and yet he is driven to give expression to his own proclivities; because of his sensitive organization he is often pulled two ways at the same time. Events having to do with his place in his society take on major significance, and he often functions best when his own ends are totally subordinate to the common end, or to the "Glory of God." Inversely, when frustrated in such efforts, or rejected by his group, the individual may seriously abreact or even die. He is jeopardized not only by those forces that threaten survival of self and kin and opportunities for procreation, but also he is endangered when through the actions of other people, his growth, development and expression of individual proclivities are blocked, and often when his esthetic needs and creative potential are not fulfilled. Further, man's lively appetite for challenge, exploration and adventure, by driving him into situations fraught with difficulty and hardship, is extremely likely to lead to frustration and enhanced vulnerability.

On the other hand, challenge for man is essential and some threat is desirable, if not necessary, for the formation of salutary adaptive reaction patterns, and thus for proper human development. However, threats to the stability of intimate human relations, and to the establishment of sustaining values, especially during the dependent years, and threats that wipe out hope and faith in man may have grave effects (35).

Particular mention should be made of stimuli stemming from sudden and violent alterations in environment that in themselves have little direct noxious effect, but because such changes alter basic and established relations between the creature and his environment they are potentially noxious, engender stress, and often evoke major reactions inappropriate in kind and amount. Such a situation is illustrated by some American Indian tribes taken from their home land and put into reservations within a few miles' distance, in essentially the same physical environment, but in a setting of social disorganization, with a resultant appalling increase in mortality from tuberculosis (36, 37). In this case, the noxious agent was the violent and sudden change which altered established human relationships; whereas light, food, sun, air, hygienic circumstances and clothing remained ostensibly unaltered, or perhaps were somewhat improved.

Also worthy of special mention, since they engender stress, are those situations, jobs for example, which, although non-noxious in themselves, are repetitious, non-challenging and monotonous. On the other hand, there is that category of excessive stimulation especially relevant to those persons whose aspirations, whose pursuit of adventure and excitement, and whose appetite for challenge exceed their capacities.

Man's special proclivity for reacting to symbols as though to significant events enhances his satisfactions, but also increases his ability to perceive threats.

The thesis to be considered in detail in these pages may be stated as follows: the stress accruing from a situation is based on large part on the way the affected subject perceives it; perception depends upon a multiplicity of factors, including the genetic equipment, basic individual needs and longings, earlier conditioning influences, and a host of life experiences and cultural pressures. No one of these can be singled out for exclusive emphasis. The common denominator of "stress disorders" is reaction to circumstances of threatening significance to the organism.

The particular adaptive pattern evoked by a noxious agent or threat is the resultant of past life experience which conditions individuals to react in specific ways. Hence "etiology" in disease becomes a function not merely of precipitating incident and setting, but largely of the past of the individual and his stock.

Much confusion has surrounded attempts to develop a concept of cause and the difficulty of distinguishing between significant forces and the mechanisms they actuate (38). All mechanisms are perforce organic and at the same time functional, since they involve the function of units of the body's equipment. The agents that activate them on the other hand, are likely to derive from the outside, often from noxious stimuli in the environment. Multiple forces may activate pathogenic mechanisms and produce bodily disorders and diseases. The ability of symbolic stimul' to participate in the activation of disease mechanisms depends upon the fact that most bodily organs are connected with, and responsive to impulses reaching them via autonomic and endocrine pathways, from the highest integrative levels of the nervous system, the interpretive areas of the brain.

The characteristics of a situation acting as a stimulus may activate, but do not determine the nature of the response. The response will depend upon the state of the organism at the time of stimulation and on the organism's genetic equipment and other inherent characteristics. Thus, a precisely similar situation may have entirely different effects on two individuals or on the same individual at different times. When visceral behavior leads to disease, the pathology represents the resultant of an algebraic equation in which the factors include inherent characteristics of the individual, the timing and other circumstances of the situation, the nature and quantity of the noxious agent or experience, and other forces, threatening or protective, acting at the same time.

Man's ability to adapt, that is to remain free of disease, depends not only on his own inherent capacities and past experience, but also on his motivation and the support and refreshment that his environment can afford him.

BIBLIOGRAPHY

1. WOLFF, H. G.: Protective reaction patterns and disease (Loeb Lecture). *Ann. Intern. Med.*, 27:955-969, 1947.
2. WOLFF, H. G.: Life situations, emotions and disease. In: *Teach-*

ing Psychotherapeutic Medicine, Cambridge, Harvard, 1947, pp. 376-379.

3. WOLFF, H. G.: Life stress and bodily disease—A formulation. *Proc. Ann. Res. Nerv. Ment. Dis., 29*:1059, 1950. *Life Stress and Bodily Disease,* Baltimore, Williams and Wilkins, 1950.

4. WOLFF, H. G.: Life stress and cardiovascular disorders. *Circulation, 1*:187, 1950.

5. PAVLOV, I.: *Conditioned Reflexes. An Investigation of the Physiological Activity of the Cerebral Cortex,* trans. by G. V. Aurep. New York, Oxford, 1927. Also: New York, Dover Publications, 1960.

6. PAVLOV, I.:*Lectures on Conditioned Reflexes,* trans. by W. H. Gantt. New York, International Publishers, 1928.

7. SELYE, H., and FORTIER, C.: Adaptive reactions to stress. *Proc. Ass. Res. Nerv., Ment. Dis., 29*:3, 1950.

8. MITTELMANN, B., and WOLFF, H. G.: Affective states and skin temperature: Experimental study of subjects with "Cold Hands" and Raynaud's Syndrome. *Psychosom. Med., 1*:271-292, 1939.

9. MAURER, EDWARD L.: *Technical Mechanics,* New York, Wiley, 1917.

10. WOLFF, H. G., WOLF, S., GRACE, W. J., HOLMES, T. H., STEVENSON, I., STRAUB, L., GOODELL, H., and SETON, P.: Changes in form and function of mucous membranes occurring as part of protective patterns in man during periods of life stress and emotional conflict. *Trans. Ass. Amer. Physicians, 61*:313-334, 1948.

11. WOLFF, H. G.: Life situations, emotions and bodily disease. In: *Feelings and Emotions, The Mooseheart Symposium.* Martin L. Reymart, Ed., New York, McGraw-Hill, 1950, Chap. 24, pp. 284-324.

12. WOLFF, H. G.: Stress, Emotions and Bodily Disease in Civil Life. Presented April 12, 1951 to the Medical Service Officer Basic Course, Army Medical Service Graduate School. Washington, D.C., Military Medicine Notes, Vol. 1, 1951.

13. WOLFF, H. G.: Stress, Emotions and Bodily Disease in Civil Life. Presented March 17, 1953, *Symposium on Stress,* Army Medical Service Graduate School, Walter Reed Army Medical Center, Washington, D.C., pp. 132-141.

14. WOLFF, H. G.: Changes in Vulnerability of Tissue: An Aspect of Man's Response to Threat. The National Institute of

Health, Annual Lectures, 1953, pp. 38-71. U.S. Dept. of Health, Education and Welfare. Publication #388.

15. HINKLE, L. E., and WOLFF, H. G.: The nature of Man's adaptation to his total environment and the relation of this to illness. *Arch. Intern Med. (Chicago)*, *99*:442-460, 1957.

16. SCHOTTSTAEDT, W. W., PINSKY, R. H., MACKLER, D., and WOLF, S: Sociologic, psychologic and metabolic observations on patients in the community of a metabolic ward. *Amer. J. Med.*, *25*:248, 1958.

17. SCHOTTSTAEDT, W. W. PINSKY, R. H., MACKLER, D., and WOLF, S.: Prestige and social interaction on a metabolic ward. *Psychosom. Med.*, *21*:131, 1959.

18. SCHOTTSTAEDT, W. W., JACKMAN, N. R., MCPHAIL, C. S., and WOLF, S.: Social interactions on a metabolic ward—the relation of problems of status to chemical balance. *J. Psychosom. Res.*, *7*:83-95, 1963.

19. SCHOTTSTAEDT, W. W., and WOLF, S.: The evaluation of psychologic factors in illness. *Med. Clin. N. Amer.*, *46*:859-864, 1962.

20. SCHOTTSTAEDT, W. W.: *Psychophysiological Approach in Medical Practice*. Chicago, Year Book Publishers, Inc., 1960.

21. STEVENSON, IAN: *Medical History Taking*. New York, Hoeber, 1960.

22. WOLFF, H. G.: Life stress and bodily disease: The nature of stress in Man. In: *Contributions Toward Medical Psychology*. Vol. 1, A. Weider, Ed. New York, Ronald, 1953, Chap. 14, pp. 315-367.

23. WOLFF, H. G.: Disease and patterns of behavior. In: *The Hour if Insight: A Sequel to Moments of Personal Discovery* from Religion and Civilization Series, R. M. McIver, Ed. New York, Harper, 1953, pp. 29-39. Also see: *Patients, Physicians and Illness*, E. Garthy Jaco, Ed. Chicago, Free Press, 1958, pp. 54-60.

24. BILISOLY, F. N., GOODELL, H., and WOLFF, H. G.: Vasodilatation, lowered pain threshold, and increased tissue vulnerability. Effects dependent upon peripheral nerve function. *Arch. Intern. Med. (Chicago)*, *94*:759-773, 1954.

25. WOLFF, H. G.: Dormant human potential. *Arch. Neurol. (Chicago)*, *6*:261-263, 1962.

26. WOLFF, H. G.: What hope does for man. Science and Humanity Section, *Saturday Review*, pp. 42-45, 1956. (Also reprinted and distributed by N. Y. State Committee on TB and P.H. and

N. Y. State Heart Assoc., Inc.) Also see: Has disease meaning? *Soc. of N.Y. Hosp. Rec.,* May 8, 1956, pp. 10-17.

27. WOLF, STEWART: A new view of disease. *Trans. Amer. Clin. Climat. Ass., 74*:168-175, 1963, and *J.A.M.A., 184(2)*:129, 1963.

28. VAIHAINGER, HANS: *The Philosophy of "As If".* Trans. C. K. Ogden, London, Routledge, 1949.

29. SIMMONS, LEO, and WOLFF, H. G.: *Social Science in Medicine.* New York, Russell Sage Foundation, 1954.

30. HALDANE, J. B. S., and PRIESTLEY, J. G.: *Respiration,* London, Oxford, 1935.

31. HINKLE, L. E., and WOLFF, H. G.: Health and Social Environment: Experimental investigations. In: *Exploration in Social Psychiatry.* Leighton, Clauson and Wilson, Eds. New York, Basic Books, 1957, Chap. IV, pp. 105-137.

32. WOLF, STEWART: Life stress and patterns of disease. In: *The Psychological Basis of Medical Practice.* Harold Lief, Victor Lief, and Nina Lief, Eds. New York, Hoeber, 1963, Chap. 9, p. 109.

33. WOLF, STEWART: *A Formulation of Psychosomatic Mechanisms,* Proc. Third World Congress of Psychiatry. Montreal, Univ. of Tronto Press, 1963.

34. WOLFF, H. G., Ed.: *Life Stress and Bodily Disease.* Proc. Ass. Res. Nerv. Ment. Dis., Vol. 29, 1949. Baltimore, Williams and Wilkins, 1950.

35. WOLFF, H. G.: The mind-body relationship. In: *An Outline of Man's Knowledge,* New York, Doubleday, 1960, Chap. 2, pp. 43-72.

36. MOORMAN, LEWIS J.: Tuberculosis on the Navaho Reservation. *Amer. Rev. Tuberc., 61*:586, 1950.

37. McDOUGAL, J. B.: *Tuberculosis—A Global Study in Social Pathology.* Baltimore, Williams and Wilkins, 1949.

38. WOLF, S.: Disease as a Way of Life. Neural Integration in Systemic Pathology. *Perspect. Biol. Med.,* Spring, 1961, pp. 288-305.

Chapter II

METHODS OF INVESTIGATION

THE RELATIONSHIP of stress and disease has been studied by Harold Wolff and those about him not only in the context of daily living but also with reference to the goals of the individual and the mores of his culture. The investigator attempts to identify among several reactions and adjustments those which are relevant to a given bodily dysfunction or disease.

SELECTION OF PATIENTS FOR STUDY

Subjects were considered suitable for experimental study when they were geographically accessible to the laboratory, reasonably articulate, and cooperative. Some of the most crucial observations were made on highly motivated patients who took pride in their participation in research (1-4). On the other hand, it was necessary to guard against selecting individuals whose personality peculiarities were related mainly to a willingness to volunteer—a distorting factor discussed by Jellinek (5). It was often useful to select subjects for special study at random from the regular population of a general medical or medical sub-specialty clinic (6-8). Thus in gathering hypertensives, for example, the request of the investigator was for referral of "run-of-the-mill" hypertensive patients and specifically not for neurotic patients who happened to have hypertension. When patients were acquired either through referral or through the regular participation of the investigator in the responsibilities of the clinic, the investigator assumed the care of the patient and only rarely studied another man's patient for whom he had no responsibility.

Private patients were also studied in considerable numbers. Very few patients of any category failed to cooperate in the experimental procedures. Indeed, most of them recognized the

13

potential value to themselves of the extra attention from their physician and interpreted the sometimes elaborate experimental procedures as evidence of an interest in them and a serious concern for their welfare.

In the course of exploration of a process, the subject most suitable for study is often one with unusual or extreme manifestations, one in whom the characteristics of the disease may be found in high concentration. Many such subjects were deliberately selected for special study. Often enough, experience with prominent manifestations in some patients enabled more subtle indications to be recognized in others.

From time to time, data unobtainable from intact human subjects were obtained through study of those with special defects or those who had undergone surgical removal of a part or other deforming procedure. Thus, information on the modulating effects of higher nervous centers on vascular reflexes was gathered through the study of subjects with complete section of the spinal cord (9, 10). Those in whom parts of the brain had been damaged or removed also lent themselves to special study (11-13); and the subject with the gastric fistula, Tom, was an abundant source of important information about reaction patterns involving the stomach over a period of nearly twenty years (1-3).

TECHNIQUES AND APPARATUS

It has frequently been pointed out in contrasting the techniques of the naturalist with those of the experimenter that any contrived arrangement for experimental purposes, however simple, introduces artifacts and allows only an approximation of the natural responses of the subject under study.* The experimenter must live with these limitations. They have been less restrictive when it has been possible to make measurements as, for example, of blood pressure, pulse or electrocardiogram by telemetering or by a portable tape recording device as a subject goes about his daily activities (14).

Many of the studies reported in this volume concern the

*Journal of Psychosomatic Research. Symposium on Measurement in Psychosomatic Research, V. 8, #3, Dec. 1964.

behavior of the skin and various mucous membranes. While it was often necessary to apply measuring devices such as thermocouples to these surfaces in order to achieve relative precision, a great deal could be learned from observations of turgor, moisture and color change. Indeed, from such data reliable inferences regarding direction and changes in blood flow could be drawn. Carefully standardized color photography was used to provide comparisons and permanent records (1, 2, 15). See Frontispiece.

At times complex devices have been employed, but because of the need in human experimentation to take advantage of fortuitous and unheralded events, the simpler the device, the better, as long as it yields reliable information concerning the function being measured.

The technical procedures used have included physical means: controlled pressures, temperatures, measurements of viscosity, and electrical resistance (16) ; biochemical studies of the blood, urine and tissue fluids; photography; mechanical and electronic recording of the movements of hollow viscera and of pulsation of vessels; and in collaboration with various specialists the highly technical instruments of the neurosurgeon (17) , the otolaryngologist, ophthalmologist and urologist, among others (18) .

In human subjects, it has been observed that uncomfortable apparatus which restricts movement and may inflict some degree of pain is accompanied by trifling alterations in the bodily indicators compared to those resulting from the subtler aspects of the experimental surroundings, the curt manner or inattentiveness of an assistant, lack of poise and assurance on the part of the experimenter, maladroit questions or awkward efforts at reassurance (19-22) .

Taking these factors into consideration and assuming the skill and poise of the experimenters it was found generally preferable to utilize apparatus which itself required relatively little "nursing" so that the experimenter's full attention could be accorded to the subject. Only thus could the nuances in the patient's responses be appreciated and utilized.

CHARACTERISTICS OF THE INVESTIGATORS

Investigators using the techniques and apparatus described were equipped both to evaluate the person and the behavior of the organ in question. Often enough, as mentioned above, the collaborative assistance of those with highly developed technical skills was obtained; but for the creative process, for the posing of a penetrating question to Nature, a broad biological (including psychological) orientation was desirable in a single person, or in a small group of investigators working and thinking in close concert. Frequently, little new knowledge is brought to light when original studies are attempted by a "team" of experts representing a variety of disciplines but not necessarily able to think and ask questions in the other fellow's area. Such "teams" may be highly productive in developing and elaborating discoveries but are rarely capable of making them.

The reach for new knowledge requires an alertness and sensitivity to cues often subtle and sometimes occurring only once in many trials. Here the skill and intuition of the explorer is indispensable to the task of picking up and following leads. Fixity of purpose requires flexibility of method and often a readiness to abandon a question, a concept or a direction for a more fruitful one. Creative imagination is perhaps the most valuable quality of the discoverer. It is important, too, that the tools of the investigator do not obscure a significant but subtle cue. Claude Bernard (23) illustrated how a statistical analysis under some circumstances can obliterate an important lead when in one animal with one picqure of the fourth ventricle he produced glycosuria and in the next nine trials failed to do so.

ASKING THE QUESTION

The most difficult part of any original research is asking the crucial question. In the case of bodily reactions to the meaningful circumstances of life, one can conceive of focussing attention on the stimulus event, on the integrative process which formulates the response, or on the effector manifestation itself. Many have held that fruitful investigation of the relationship of life stress to bodily disease must await methods of quantifying "emotion" or of precise measurement of symbolic stimuli. Thus, many investigators have made heroic efforts to provide a "standard stimulus" for their subjects. Actually, it is not difficult to quantify the input. It is possible to call an individual a coward in a precisely modulated tone so that the decibels may be accurately measured and hence the energy transmitted through the ear drum and the middle ear to the organ of Corti is as nicely quantitated as any stimulus in biological research. Such pains at quantification, however, would not reward the investigator with a uniformity of response from person to person or even from time to time in the same person. Energy fed via receptors into the nervous system actuates an integrative process which ultimately interprets the event in the light of individual proclivities and past experience as threatening, neutral, or pleasurable and to what degree. Thus the stimulus gains its force. It would appear, therefore, that the search for the "standard stimulus" is a search for the will-o'-the-wisp (24). The important concern is more the relevance than the quantity of a stimulus situation. It may be illuminating to recall that the identification of micro-organisms as agents of disease depend little on quantifying the number of microbes to which an individual was exposed, but rather on the susceptibility of the individual to develop the disease in addition to the capability of the organism in whatever quantity to produce the disease (25-29).

Nowadays, students of infectious disease recognize that the presence of the micro-organism, however indispensable, is not sufficient as the cause of illness (30, 31). The crucial question at present appears to be the way in which the host handles the invasion. In other words, it is his vulnerability. Susceptibility and resistance then (32), depend not alone on interaction between host and parasite, but also on precipitating factors, as is further discussed in Chapter IV.

In relating life stress to disease, the most promising area of study up to the present, as pointed out in the W H O report on stress and disease (33, 34), has been the efferent manifestation, the organ changes resulting from the output of the central nervous system dependent in turn on the integrative process (31). The rapid expansion of knowledge of interactions within the brain may make it possible within the foreseeable future to direct inquiries at the integrative process. In the meantime, however, there is still much to be learned on the output side and in relating the output to the nature of the stimulus-input (35, 36).

With the last objective in mind, a bodily disturbance or disorder has been considered capable of approach when an indicator of its presence and of variations in its activity has been accessible to observation, and hopefully measurable and recordable.

INTERPRETATION OF THE SUBJECTS' PERCEPTIONS AND ATTITUDES

In order to correlate bodily changes with a subject's reactions to his experiences, it is necessary to understand the personality of the individual as thoroughly as possible (37-39).

Some workers have preferred to restrict the study of the person to data derived from free association, dreams, and from the analysis of the relationship between the individual and his physician (40-46). In the studies reported in this volume, such data have been included but in addition other information about the life history of the individual in his cultural framework was gathered. Special attention was accorded the social situation of the subject in relation to his job, his associates at and away from work, and his community. Education, family background, his general intelligence, talents and proclivities, and the "mobility" of his social position were seen as important contributory data. So were the demands, values, standards and actions of the parents, siblings, spouses and "superiors." Also explored were the preferences and prejudices of the group with which the subject was or wished to be identified.

Figure 1 illustrates the way in which the data from the life history of the patient could be correlated with symptoms and manifestations of disease.

Historical data were supplemented by data from the subject's statements, from his appearance, dress, manner of speaking, gestures, posture; from his reactions in the company of others including the physician, authoritative figures, associates, competitors and subordinates; from his dreams and associations and things said and left unsaid. The kind of relationship the patient

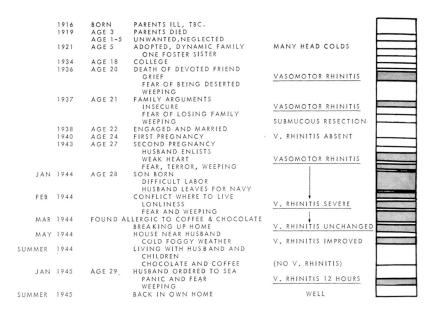

1916	BORN	PARENTS ILL, TBC.	
1919	AGE 3	PARENTS DIED	
	AGE 1-5	UNWANTED,NEGLECTED	
1921	AGE 5	ADOPTED, DYNAMIC FAMILY	MANY HEAD COLDS
		ONE FOSTER SISTER	
1934	AGE 18	COLLEGE	
1936	AGE 20	DEATH OF DEVOTED FRIEND	
		GRIEF	VASOMOTOR RHINITIS
		FEAR OF BEING DESERTED	
		WEEPING	
1937	AGE 21	FAMILY ARGUMENTS	
		INSECURE	VASOMOTOR RHINITIS
		FEAR OF LOSING FAMILY	
		WEEPING	SUBMUCOUS RESECTION
1938	AGE 22	ENGAGED AND MARRIED	
1940	AGE 24	FIRST PREGNANCY	V. RHINITIS ABSENT
1943	AGE 27	SECOND PREGNANCY	
		HUSBAND ENLISTS	
		WEAK HEART	VASOMOTOR RHINITIS
		FEAR, TERROR, WEEPING	
JAN 1944	AGE 28	SON BORN	
		DIFFICULT LABOR	
		HUSBAND LEAVES FOR NAVY	
FEB 1944		CONFLICT WHERE TO LIVE	
		LONLINESS	V. RHINITIS SEVERE
		FEAR AND WEEPING	
MAR 1944		FOUND ALLERGIC TO COFFEE & CHOCOLATE	
		BREAKING UP HOME	V. RHINITIS UNCHANGED
MAY 1944		HOUSE NEAR HUSBAND	
		COLD FOGGY WEATHER	V. RHINITIS IMPROVED
SUMMER 1944		LIVING WITH HUSBAND AND	
		CHILDREN	
		CHOCOLATE AND COFFEE	(NO V. RHINITIS)
JAN 1945	AGE 29	HUSBAND ORDERED TO SEA	
		PANIC AND FEAR	V. RHINITIS 12 HOURS
		WEEPING	
SUMMER 1945		BACK IN OWN HOME	WELL

Figure 1. Life chart illustrating coincidence of situational threats and nasal disturbances in an insecure, anxious woman. The black bars at the right indicate the occurrence, duration and intensity of troublesome symptoms.

attempted to establish with the physician was evaluated. Analysis of the stream of talk was particularly helpful when there was blocking, self-contradiction, irony, hyperbole or non-sequitur. Such data were supplemented by a variety of psychometric and word and picture association tests. In studies of children, their play with toys was observed. From these sources and from statements by friends or members of the family the trained observer attempted an appraisal of personality and reaction patterns of the patient with which he correlated fluctuations in the course of the illness in question.

Intimate knowledge of the habits and ways of life of numbers of subjects with the variety of disease under study may reveal a similarity among them. Common patterns of mood, thought and behavior could be recognized among sufferers from a particular bodily disorder or disease. A notable example is in the personality features of persons with migraine headaches. Often not delineated in formal psychological testing, the common features such as perfectionism, inflexibility, feelings of insecurity, and resentment were nevertheless recognizable in attitudes, ways of expression, characteristic behavior in certain situations and in relationships with others. Such constellations of personality reactions were often predictable and after repeated interviews frequently became evident to the patients themselves who at first had denied the characteristics and had consciously or unconsciously concealed them more or less effectively in their superficial behavior, and particularly in response to questionnaires (4, 38).

DIARIES

A helpful device for the study of recurring attitudes and emotions in reaction to day-to-day events was the diary. Patients were asked to record each day's events and their reactions to them, including symptoms, and in addition to make an estimate on a percentage scale of their efficiency of performance for the day. Patients with vascular headache of the migraine type were found to be particularly conscientious in keeping diaries, but most subjects were willing to cooperate to some extent in this task. Sometimes the information recorded gave a clear picture of the build-up of tension over a period of days and pin-pointed an event with precipitation and exacerbation of symptoms (4, 6).

Often enough, the events recorded each day gave little intrinsic information, but nevertheless provided at times unique and valuable leads for exploratory discussion. Therefore, the diaries were reviewed periodically with the patient in an attempt to analyse the significance of the recorded material and to elicit further significant data. In conjunction with the diary method, the use of check lists, such as feelings, hours of sleep, and estimations of energy and efficiency was helpful, especially in revealing states of conflict, frustration or depression. The questionnaire method was useful for screening large numbers of men and women, and for detecting emotional disorders in patients presenting themselves with defined, or ill defined complaints. The data from questionnaires often times suggested the kind of situation and interpersonal relationship pertinent to an individual patient's symptoms and bodily changes, leading to recognition of specific topics which will evoke the protective reactions involved (47, 48).

Interestingly, since the percentage estimate of efficiency seemed to be a relatively neutral commitment patients responded with considerable candor and indirectly revealed their prevailing degree of anxiety and conflict. Diaries also afforded helpful information when certain recurring events were found to be predictably associated with exacerbation of symptoms either on the day of the event or on immediately succeeding ones. In the early analysis of the diary with the patient, it may not have been possible to elicit any hint of conflict in connection with the event or the persons concerned, but after repeated documentation of an association of events and symptoms the conflict could often be brought to the surface.

"STRESS INTERVIEWS"

When temporal correlations were possible between certain prototype life experiences and the bodily changes being measured, further evidence was sought in an experimental setting. After a control period during which the patient was lightly diverted and made comfortable and while the indicators in question were being recorded, a "stress interview" was begun. The procedure consisted of introducing as a topic for discussion the circumstances which had been found to correlate with the bodily disturbance. The interviewer's manner was usually neither hostile nor critical but rather quizzical and often skeptical. He tried to manage the relationship so that it was not necessary for him to talk very much. Instead, he listened intently, prompting the subject and bringing him back to the primary topic when he strayed away from it. In a successful interview of this type, it was possible to rivet the subject's attention on his troubles, and to observe an intense "re-living" type of reaction in him for twenty minutes to an hour, and thus to elicit the sought-for bodily change. Through such a maneuver, the evidence of a linkage between the topic of conflict and the bodily change was considered strengthened.

Finally, every attempt was made to obliterate the exacerbated reaction and to restore the situation which prevailed during the control period by an alteration in the manner of the interviewer. He suddenly abandoned his skepticism, manifested complete understanding of the patient's circumstances and offered his full emotional support. As he appeared to be successful in restoring the patient's serenity, he resumed the lightly diverting conversation of the control period. When by such efforts it was possible to "turn off" the observed bodily change, a further confirmation of the original hypothesis had been achieved. It was not necessary under these circumstances to infer that the specific topic was relevant to the disease or indeed that it was of necessity the main focus of the patient's problems of adjustment. However, it could be assumed that the topic evoking the protective reaction *was representative of the kind of situation and interpersonal relationship* pertinent to the subject's symptoms and bodily changes. By further detailed study, it was then sometimes possible to establish which features were of most basic dynamic significance to the patient (49-68).

CONSCIOUS AND UNCONSCIOUS INTEGRATIVE PROCESSES AND EMOTION

The concept of the unconscious has helped greatly in the understanding of mental processes, including their relevance to bodily disorders. Whether or not the subject is actually aware of the significance of the situation or, indeed, even altogether sensible to the experience itself does not necessarily determine the nature or extent of the reaction, except as will, desire, or motivation add to the picture. The usefulness of the idea of unconscious processes has been hampered by certain misconceptions, however, such as the naive implication that the "unconscious" occupies a place in the brain. Perhaps just as unsophisticated is the notion that unconscious motivations or purposes differ from other neural activity occurring at the highest integrative levels.

A great deal of evaluative function occurs in the brain of men without awareness, and, of course, even during sleep. Witness the fact that a mother may awaken to the faint cry of an infant but sleep through a much louder noise which has no important meaning to her. Unconscious mental activity may, indeed, be much more precise than that undertaken during awareness. A fully alert man may miss by an hour or more in judging the time of day and yet discipline himself to awaken within a minute of a set time (68).

Important emotional conflicts are likely to be shunted out of awareness for the general comfort of the individual. The information remains in the brain, however, perfectly capable of being recruited on appropriate stimulation and of entering the complex process of behavior. Thus, emotional responses may be aroused, such as fear, anxiety or resentment, with or without awareness of the original conflict. Responses may also be formulated with or without awareness of the stimulus and with or without an emotion or feeling state. These may be in terms of striving, creating, destroying, avoidance, and other patterns of behavior.

The frequent association of manifestations of physiological dysfunction with overt emotional disturbance has led to the widely accepted but confusing proposition that emotions are the cause of bodily reactions. The confusion is further compounded by the difficulty of defining an emotion. Different writers use the term in different ways. Literally, the word implies movement of some sort. Thus, an emotion is clearly a manifestation, not a cause. Many authors, however, equate the term with a feeling state. To them, an emotion is a sort of sensation or at least an awareness which may be pleasant or unpleasant; for example, joy, satisfaction, hope, and appetite fall into the category of emotions. But again emotion is part of the reaction to some circumstance which is pleasing, frightening, or frustrating, not the cause of the reaction. Finally, some workers apply the term emotion to conscious or unconscious mental processes whereby events are interpreted in view of personality and past experience. In this instance, as already discussed, neural connections are made because of the significance of the event but without the process necessarily being brought to awareness. An emotion viewed in this light would constitute an essential part

of the neural integrative activity and, thus, part of the mechanism
of response, but it still would not be the cause. An emotion,
therefore, may be looked upon variously as: (a) a manifestation
or part of the reaction pattern aroused as a consequence of the
interpretation of a life experience; (b) a feeling state occurring
because of the conscious or unconscious interpretation of a life
experience, or (c) an often repressed but functioning aspect
of the interpretation of a life experience. In any case, bodily
changes appear to derive from the individual's evaluation of his
experience, consciously or unconsciously, and with or without
overt emotional expression.

ESTABLISHMENT OF CONTROLS

Control Subjects: The nature of the control needed in an
experimental situation varied with the question being asked.
In establishing characteristics typical of a certain entity as for
instance hypertension, it was convenient to compare the hypertensive subjects with a group of patients with asthma and a
group of presumably healthy persons matched as closely as
possible for age, sex, education and work experience. In demonstrating the pertinence of a conflict situation to a particular
bodily reaction, it was more suitable for each subject to act as
his own control.

Control Procedures: In the short term experiments utilizing
"stress interview" and other procedures, the validity of inferences
from the changes observed during the stimulus period depended
in large measure on the adequacy of control periods before and
after.

In setting the length of an experimental session, the investigator must balance the need for control periods of adequate
length before and after the experimental procedure against his
awareness of the fact that tension and boredom associated with
long sessions may distort the findings.

Van der Valk and Groen (16) have demonstrated that
forced inactivity in the experimental setting may in itself produce profound effects on some patients. Pavlov (69, 70) emphasized this to be important in certain dogs. Long delays

between phases of stimulation, too often repeated stimuli, or protracted restraint in the experimental harness, made difficult the interpretation of the subsequent reaction to specific experimental stimuli. Scott (71), Liddell (72, 73), and Gantt (74, 75) have repeatedly confirmed these observations. In order to assess the effects of boredom and tension in a long session, or when it was necessary for the experiment to be relatively short, it was helpful to match each experiment with a control session on another day during which the appropriate indicators were measured throughout but no stress-evoking stimuli were knowingly introduced.

REPRODUCIBILITY OF REACTION PATTERNS

In any experimental work, the ability to replicate a finding is important. With the methods of study described above, a replication in kind and amount can often but not always be achieved. Some individuals respond in a predictably uniform way when placed in similar situations. In others, repetition seems to "desensitize" so that their response becomes less and less evident. In the same individual, it appears that some stimuli, especially those having great symbolic importance may not lose their power to evoke reactions while those having less symbolic significance often rapidly lose their capacity to evoke bodily changes.

A rapid decline of brain wave responses to a given topic of discussion when repeated has been noted in a wide variety of experiments with the encephalogram (52). The rate of decline varies with many factors. The decline of wave responses with repetition of stimulus may be noted whether the stimulus is a suggestion given during hypnosis or discussion of a symptom-provoking life situation. If the stimulus or problem acquires deeper significance with each repetition, however, response may not diminish but may even become accentuated. Also, variations in feeling state may be associated with variable responses to a standard stimulus (76-78).

The phenomenon of dwindling response was carefully analyzed by Furer and Hardy while changes in skin resistance in reaction to noxious stimulation were being recorded (79). It was shown that pain of moderate intensity induced by thermal stimulation was associated with a fall in skin resistance of the palms during initial trials; but as the stimulus was repeatedly presented, the psychogalvanic skin response became less and less, even though the intensity of pain experienced was unaltered. With pain of high intensity, however, such dwindling of effect did not occur. Also, if the stimuli which were producing no reaction because of this dwindling effect were withheld for a week and then reapplied, they again called forth responses for periods of varying duration.

ECOLOGICAL APPROACH

During the past century, epidemiological studies contributed widely to our understanding of the pathogenesis of infectious diseases. Recently, the scope of epidemiology has been broadened to include not only the interactions of host and invading parasite but also significant interactions of man with a wide variety of noxious forces in his environment (80-84, 25, 31, 6, 26-30, 85-95). Concepts of disease have also been enlarged. No longer does the restrictive view prevail that the word disease encompasses only visceral disturbances and involuntary experiences (91-93). As obesity, the result of voluntary behavior became recognized as a disease (96, 97), so did alcoholism (98) and drug addiction (99). Now, many behavioral deviations including antisocial behavior and suicide are recognized as manifestations of disease. Indeed, the ecological setting and social forces which are associated with the prevalence of suicide have been nicely documented (100-102).

Methods have been greatly refined and supplemented by techniques from other disciplines such as social anthropology (123, 103-112) so that reliable data may be gathered across the broad spectrum of health and disease. The past fifteen years has seen the rapid accumulation of data on the comparative prevalence in widely distant parts of the world of diseases such as atherosclerosis (113-119), hypertension, rheumatic heart disease, metabolic disorders (120, 121) and various forms of cancer (122,

123). Such studies seem likely to illuminate the possible relevance of cultural and social as well as genetic, dietary, climatic and meteorological forces to pathogenic processes. Populations have either been studied *in situ* or after displacement; as still relatively homogenous groups they have been studied in their new locality and compared to the indigenous population (124-129).

Adequate application of the ecological approach to problems of life stress and bodily disease is difficult and demanding. The approach must also include the careful study of individuals and the measurement and recording of their patterns of bodily reaction. In short, all of the methodology which can add precision to the study of disease in man must be used. Progress in the future will require equal emphasis on breadth of study of the group, and depth of study of the individual. Careful attention to each of these vectors should ultimately lead to clarification of the central question as to what motivates a person to select one course of action or pattern of reaction over another. Other age-old questions may be brought closer to solution, such as whether or not or to what degree temperament is inherited and if, and to what degree in man, learned behavior can be incorporated into the genetic code.

BIBLIOGRAPHY

1. WOLF, S, and WOLFF, H. G.: *Human Gastric Function—An Experimental Study of a Man and His Stomach,* New York, Oxford, 1943, and 1947.
2. WOLF, S.: *The Stomach.* New York, Oxford, 1966.
3. WOLF, S.: The final studies of Tom. *Trans. Amer. Clin. Climat. Ass., 71*:159-165, 1959.
4. WOLFF, H. G.: *Headache and Other Head Pain.* New York, Oxford, 1948, and 1963.
5. JELLINEK, E. M.: Clinical tests on comparative effectiveness of analgesic drugs. *Biometrics, 2*:87-91, 1946.
6. WOLF, S., CARDON, P., SHEPARD, E., and WOLFF, H. G.: *Life Stress and Essential Hypertension.* Baltimore, Williams and Wilkins, 1955.
7. WOLF, STEWART, and WOLFF, H. G.: A summary of experimental

evidence relating life stress to the pathogenesis of essential hypertension in man. In: *Hypertension: Symposium,* University of Minnesota, Sept., 1950. Minneapolis, Univ. Minnesota Press, 1951, pp. 288-330.

8. WOLFF, H. G., WOLF, S., in collaboration with B. B. Berle, H. S. Ripley, W. H. Dunn and E. M. Shepard: The Management of Hypertensive Patients. In: *Hypertension, A Symposium,* E. T. Bell, Ed. Minneapolis, Univ. Minnesota Press, 1951.

9. BERLIN, L., GUTHRIE, T. C., GOODELL, H., and WOLFF, H. G.: Analysis of the reflex function of the isolated spinal cord using measured stimuli. *Trans. Amer. Neurol. Ass.,* 1952, pp. 106-110.

10. BERLIN, L., GUTHRIE, T. C., GOODELL, H., and WOLFF, H. G.: Studies on the central excitatory state. 1. Factors responsible for the variability of the motor response to cutaneous stimulation in human subjects with isolated spinal cords. *Arch. Neurol. Psychiat.,* 72:764-779, 1954.

11. DOIG, R. K., WOLF, S., and WOLFF, H. G.: Study of gastric function in a "Decorticate" man with gastric fistula. *Trans. Amer. Neurol. Ass.,* 1953, pp. 239-241, and *Gastroenterology,* 23:40-44, 1953.

12. CHAPMAN, L., and WOLFF, H. G.: Studies in human cerebral function: Adaptive capacity after loss of hemisphere tissue. *Trans. Amer. Neurol. Ass.,* 1956, pp. 175-178.

13. CHAPMAN, L., and WOLFF, H. G.: The cerebral hemispheres and the highest integrative functions of man. *Arch. Neurol. (Chicago), I:*357-424, 1959.

14. HINKLE, L. E., JR., CARVER, S., BENJAMIN, B., CHRISTENSON, W. N., and STRONG, B. W.: Studies in ecology of coronary heart disease. I. Variations in the human electrocardiogram under conditions of daily life. *Arch. Environ. Health (Chicago), 9:*14-20, 1964.

15. HOLMES, T. H., GOODELL, H., WOLF, S., and WOLFF, H. G.: *The Nose: An Experimental Study of Reactions Within the Nose in Human Subjects.* Springfield, Thomas, 1950.

16. VAN DER VALK, J. M., and GROEN, J.: An investigation of the electrical resistance of the skin during induced emotional stress in normal individuals and in patients with internal disease. *Proc. Ass. Res. Nerv. Ment. Dis., 29:*279, 1950.

17. RAY, B. S., and CONSOLE, A. D.: Bodily adjustments in man

during stress in the absence of most visceral afferents and sympathetic nervous system regulation. *Proc. Ass. Res. Nerv. Ment. Dis., 29*:114, 1950.

18. WOLFF, H. G., Ed.: *Pain. Proc. Ann. Res. Nerv. Ment. Dis.,* Vol. 23, Baltimore, Williams and Wilkins, 1943.

19. PFEIFFER, J. B., JR., and WOLFF, H. G.: Studies in renal circulation during periods of life stress and accompanying emotional reactions in subjects with and without essential hypertension; observations on the role of neural activity in regulation of renal blood flow. *Proc. Ass. Res. Nerv. Ment. Dis., 29*:929, 1950. Also: *J. Clin. Invest., 29*:1227, 1950.

20. BOGDONOFF, M. D., BREHM, L., BOCK, K.: The effect of the experimenter's role upon the subject's response to an unpleasant task. *J. Psychosom. Res., 8*:137, 1964.

21. GROEN, J. J.: Methodology of psychosomatic research. *J. Psychosom. Res., 5*:12, 1960.

22. IKEMI, Y., OKONOGI, K., DOBETA, H., and HONDA, T.: Psychosomatic research in Japan. *J. Psychosom. Res., 5*:42, 1960.

23. BERNARD, CLAUDE: *Leçons sur les Propriétés Physiologiques et les Altérations Pathologiques des Liquides de l'Organisme.* Paris, Bailleurs, 1859.

24. WOLF, S.: A note on the cause of disease. *Amer. J. Med., 16*:769, 1954.

25. McDOUGAL, J. B.: *Tuberculosis—A Global Study in Social Pathology.* Baltimore, Williams and Wilkins, 1949.

26. KRAUSE, ALLEN K.: Factors in the pathogenesis of tuberculosis. *Amer. Rev. Tuberc., 18*:208, 1928.

27. KRAUSE, ALLEN K.: Tuberculosis and public health. *Amer. Rev. Tuberc., 18*:271, 1928.

28. DUBOS, R. J.: Biological and social aspects of tuberculosis. *Bull. N. Y. Acad. Med., 27*:351, 1951.

29. DUBOS, R. J.: The tubercle bacillus and tuberculosis. *Amer. Sci., 37*:353, 1949.

30. HINKLE, L. E., CHRISTENSON, W. N., BENJAMIN, B., KANE, F. D., PLUMMER, NORMAN, and WOLFF, H. G.: Observations on the role of nasal adaptive reactions, emotions and life situations in the genesis of minor respiratory illnesses. Presented, Amer. Psychosom. Soc., April, 1962. Presented to Staff, Survey Research Center, University of Michigan, Ann Arbor, November, 1964.

31. WOLF, S.: Disease as a Way of Life. Neural Integration in

Systemic Pathology. *Perspect. Biol. Med.*, pp. 288-305, Spring, 1961.

32. BAKKE, J. L., and WOLFF, H. G.: Life situations and serum antibody titers. *Psychosom. Med., 10*:327, 1948.

33. CHARVAT, J., DELL, P., and FOLKOW, BJORN: Mental factors and cardiovascular diseases. *Cardiologia (Basel), 44*:124-41, 1964.

34. *Psychosomatic Disorders:* WHO, 13th Report of the Expert Committee on Mental Health, Geneva, 1964. WHO Technical Report Series No. 275.

35. WOLF, S.: Asking the question. *Psychosom. Med., 24*:417, 1962.

36. FERNEL, J.: In: *Man on His Nature.* Sir Charles Sherrington, Ed., London, Cambridge Univ. Press, 1951.

37. WOLFF, H. G., Ed.: *Life Stress and Bodily Disease.* Proc. Ass. Res. Nerv. Ment. Dis., Vol. 29, 1949. Baltimore, Williams and Wilkins, 1950.

38. WOLFF, H. G.: Personality features and reactions of patients with migraine. *Arch. Neurol. Psychiat., 37*:895-921, 1937.

39. MITTELMAN, B., and WOLFF, H. G.: Emotions and gastroduodenal function: Experimental studies on patients with gastritis, duodenitis and peptic ulcer. *Psychosom. Med., 4*:5-61, 1942.

40. HIGGINS, J., LEDERER, H., and ROSENBAUM, M.: Life situations, emotions and idiopathic epilepsy. *Proc. Ann. Res. Nerv. Ment. Dis., 29*:137, 1950.

41. PERSKY, H., GRINKER, R. R., MIRSKY, J. A., and GAMM, S. R.: Life situations, emotions and the excretion of hippuric acid in anxiety states. *Proc. Ass. Res. Nerv. Ment. Dis., 29*:297, 1950.

42. HAM, G. C., ALEXANDER, F. G., and CARMICHAEL, H. T.: Dynamic aspects of the personality features and reactions characteristic of patients with Grave's disease. *Proc. Ass. Res. Nerv. Ment. Dis., 29*:451, 1950.

43. MIRSKY, I. A., KAPLAN, S., and BROH-KAHN, R. H.: Pepsinogen excretion (Uropepsin) as an index of the influence of various life situations on gastric secretion. *Proc. Ass. Res. Nerv. Ment. Dis., 29*:628, 1950.

44. MARGOLIN, S. G., ORRINGER, D., KAUFMAN, M. R., WINKELSTEIN, A., HOLLANDER, F., JANOWITZ, H., STEIN, A., and LEVY, M. H.: Variations of gastric functions during conscious and unconscious conflict states. *Proc. Ass. Res. Nerv. Ment. Dis., 29*:656, 1950.

45. SZASZ, T. S.: Psychosomatic aspects of salivary activity. 1. Hypersalivation in patients with peptic ulcer. *Proc. Ass. Res. Nerv. Ment. Dis., 29*:647, 1950.

46. LINDEMANN, E.: Modifications in the course of ulcerative colitis in relationship to changes in life situations and reaction patterns. *Proc. Ass. Res. Nerv. Ment. Dis., 29*:706, 1950.

47. BRODMAN, K., ERDMANN, A. J., JR., LORGE, I., GERSHENSON, C. P., and WOLFF, H. G.: Cornell Medical Index Health Questionnaire, III. The evaluation of emotional disturbances. *J. Clin. Psychol., 13*:119, 1952.

48. BRODMAN, K., ERDMANN, A. J., JR., LORGE, I., DEUTSCHBERGER, J., and WOLFF, H. G.: The Cornell Medical Index-Health Questionnaire. The predictions of psychosomatic and psychiatric disabilities in army training. *Amer. J. Psychiat., 3*:37-40, 1954.

49. HETZEL, BASIL S., GRACE, W. J., and WOLFF, H. G.: General metabolic changes during stressful life experience. *J. Psychosom. Res., 1*:186-202, 1956.

50. GRAHAM, DAVID, T.: The pathogenesis of hives: Experimental study of life situations, emotions and cutaneous vascular reactions. *Proc. Ass. Res. Nerv. Ment. Dis., 29*:987, 1950.

51. FLYNN, J. T., KENNEDY, M. A. K., and WOLF, S.: Essential hypertension in one of identical twins. An experimental study of cardiovascular reactions in the Y twins. *Proc. Ass. Res. Nerv. Ment. Dis., 29*:954, 1950.

52. BARKER, W., and BARKER, S.: Experimental production of human convulsive brain potentials by stress induced effects upon neural integrative function: Dynamics of the convulsive reaction to stress. *Proc. Ass. Res. Nerv. Ment. Dis., 29*:90, 1950.

53. HINKLE, L. E., and WOLF, S.: Studies in diabetes mellitus: Changes in glucose, ketones and water metabolism during stress. *Proc. Ass. Res. Nerv. Ment. Dis., 29*:338, 1950. Also: *J. Clin. Invest., 29*:754, 1950.

54. GOODELL, H., GRAHAM, D. T., and WOLFF, H. G.: Changes in body heat regulation associated with varying life situations and emotional states. *Proc. Ass. Res. Nerv. Ment. Dis., 29*:418, 1950.

55. RIPLEY, H. S., and WOLFF, H. G.: Life situations, emotions and glaucoma. *Proc. Ass. Res. Nerv. Ment. Dis., 29*:523, 1950. Also: *Psychosom. Med., 12*:215-224, 1950.

56. WOLF, S., and MESSIER, P. E.: Corneal vascular changes in association with conflict in a patient with phlyctenular keratitis. *Proc. Ass. Res. Nerv. Ment. Dis., 29*:537, 1950.

57. HOLMES, T. H., TREUTING, T., and WOLFF, H. G.: Life situations, emotions and nasal disease: Evidence on summative effects exhibited in patients with hay fever. *Proc. Ass. Res. Nerv. Ment. Dis., 29*:545, 1950. Also: *Psychosom. Med., 13*:71, 1951.

58. WILLARD, H. N., SWAN, R. C., JR., and WOLF, G. A., JR.: Life situations, emotions and dyspnea. *Proc. Ass. Res. Nerv. Ment. Dis., 29*:583, 1950.

59. STEVENSON, I.: Variations in the secretion of bronchial mucus during periods of life stress. *Proc. Ass. Res. Nerv. Ment. Dis., 29*:596, 1950.

60. MARCUSSEN, R. M.: Vascular headache experimentally induced by presentation of pertinent life experience. Modification of the course of vascular headache by alterations of situations and reactions. *Proc. Ass. Res. Nerv. Ment. Dis., 29*:609, 1950.

61. WOLF, S., and GLASS, G. B. J.: Correlation of conscious and unconscious conflicts with changes in gastric function and structure. Observations on the relation of the constituents of the gastric juice to the integrity of the mucous membrane. *Proc. Ass. Res. Nerv. Ment. Dis., 29*:665, 1950.

62. PRUGH, D. G.: Variations in attitudes, behavior and feeling states as exhibited in the play of children during modification in the course of ulcerative colitis. *Proc. Ass. Res. Nerv. Ment. Dis., 29*:692, 1950.

63. HOLMES, T. H., and WOLFF, H. G.: Life situations, emotions and backache. *Psychosom. Med., 14*:18-33, 1952.

64. STEVENSON, I., and DUNCAN, C. H.: Alterations in cardiac function and circulatory efficiency during periods of life stress as shown by changes in the rate, rhythm, electrocardiographic pattern and output of the heart in those with cardiovascular disease. *Proc. Ass. Ass. Res. Nerv. Ment. Dis., 29*:799, 1950.

65. SCHNEIDER, R. A.: The relation of stress to clotting time, relative viscosity and certain other biophysical alterations of the blood in the normotensive and hypertensive subjects. *Proc. Ass. Res. Nerv. Ment. Dis., 29*:818, 1950.

66. WOLF, S., and SHEPARD, E. M.: An appraisal of factors that evoke and modify the hypertensive reaction pattern. *Proc. Ass. Res. Nerv. Ment. Dis., 29*:976, 1950.

67. STRAUB, L. R., RIPLEY, H. S., and WOLF, S.: Disturbances of bladder function associated with emotional states. *Proc. Ass. Res. Nerv. Ment. Dis., 29*:1227, 1950.

68. WOLF, S.: Emotions and disease. *Physiol. for Physicians.* Vol. 1, No. 2., 1963.

69. PAVLOV, I.: *Conditioned Reflexes. An Investigation of the Physiological Activity of the Cerebral Cortex.* Trans. by G. V. Aurep. New York, Oxford, 1927. Also: New York, Dover Publications, 1960.

70. PAVLOV, I.: *Lectures on Conditioned Reflexes.* Trans. by W. H. Gantt. New York, International Publishers, 1928.

71. SCOTT, J. P.: The relative importance of social and hereditary factors in producing disturbances in life adjustment during periods of stress in laboratory animals. *Proc. Ass. Res. Nerv. Ment. Dis., 29*:61, 1950.

72. LIDDELL, H. S.: Some specific factors that modify tolerance for environmental stress. *Proc. Ass. Res. Nerv. Ment. Dis., 29*:155, 1950.

73. LIDDELL, HOWARD S.: *Emotional Hazards in Animal and Man.* Springfield, Thomas, 1956.

74. GANTT, W. H.: Disturbances in sexual functions during periods of stress. *Proc. Ass. Res. Nerv. Ment. Dis., 29*:1030, 1950.

75. GANTT, W. H.: *Experimental Basis for Neurotic Behavior.* New York, Hoeber, 1944.

76. FUNKENSTEIN, D. H.: Variations in response to standard amounts of chemical agents during alterations in feeling states in relation to occurrence of asthma. *Proc. Ass. Res. Nerv. Ment. Dis., 29*:566, 1950.

77. WOLF, S.: Cardiovascular reactions to symbolic stimuli. *Circulation, 18*:287-292, 1958.

78. WOLF, S.: The pharmacology of placebos. *Pharmacol. Rev., 11*:689-704, 1959.

79. FURER, M., and HARDY, J. D.: The reaction to pain as determined by the galvanic skin response. *Proc. Ass. Res. Nerv. Ment. Dis., 29*:72, 1950.

80. WOLFF, H. G.: Disease and patterns of behavior. In: *The Hour of Insight: A Sequel to Moments of Personal Discovery,* from Religion and Civilization Series, R. M. McIver, Ed. New York, Harper, 1953, pp. 29-39. Also see: *Patients, Physicians and Illness,* E. Garthy Jaco, Ed. Chicago, Free Press, 1958, pp. 54-60.

81. HINKLE, L. E., and WOLFF, H. G.: Health and social environment: Experimental investigations. In: *Exploration in Social Psychiatry*, Leighton, Clauson and Wilson, Eds. New York, Basic Books, 1957, Chap. IV, pp. 105-137.

82. WOLF, S.: Life stress and patterns of disease. In: *The Psychological Basis of Medical Practice*, Harold Lief, Victor Lief, and Nina Lief, Eds. New York, Hoeber, 1963, Chap. 9, p. 109.

83. WOLF, S.: *A Formulation of Psychosomatic Mechanisms*. Proc. Third World Congress of Psychiatry. Montreal, Univ. Toronto Press, 1963.

84. MOORMAN, LEWIS J.: Tuberculosis on the Navaho Reservation. *Amer. Rev. Tuberc., 61*:586, 1950.

85. HINKLE, L. E., CHRISTENSON, W. N., KANE, F. D., OSTFELD, A., THETFORD, W. N., and WOLFF, H. G.: An investigation of the relation between life experience, personality characteristics, and general susceptibility to illness. *Psychosom. Med., 20*:278-295, 1958.

86. HINKLE, L. E., JR., and PLUMMER, NORMAN: Life stress and industrial absenteeism. The concentration of illness and absenteeism in one segment of a working population. *Industr. Med. Surg., 21*:363, 1952.

87. WOLFF, H. G.: A concept of disease in man. *Psychosom. Med., 24*:25-30, 1962.

88. HINKLE, L. E., JR., and WOLFF, H. G.: Ecologic investigations of the relationship between illness, life experiences and the social environment. *Ann. Intern. Med., 49*:1373-1388, 1958.

89. HINKLE, J. E., JR., and WOLF, S.: A summary of experimental evidence relating life stress to diabetes mellitus. *J. Mount Sinai Hosp. N. Y., 19*:537-570, 1952.

90. WOLFF, H. G.: Stress and adaptive patterns resulting in tissue damage in man. *Med. Clin. N. Amer., 39*:783-797, 1955.

91. WOLFF, H. G.: Stressors as a cause of disease in man. Disorganization of behavior in man. In: *Stress and Psychiatric Disorder*, J. M. Tanner, Ed. Oxford, Blackwell, 1960, Chap. 2, pp. 17-31.

92. CHAPMAN, L., HINKLE, L. E., JR., and WOLFF, H. G.: Human ecology, disease and schizophrenia. *Amer. J. Psychiat., 117*: 193-204, 1960.

93. CHAPMAN, L., THETFORD, W. N., BERLIN, L., GUTHRIE, T., and WOLFF, H. G.: Highest integrative functions in man during stress. Chap. XXI In: *The Brain and Human Behavior,*

Baltimore, Williams and Wilkins. *Proc. Ass. Res. Nerv. Ment. Dis.*, *36*:491-534, 1958.

94. HINKLE, L. E., JR., REDMONT, R., PLUMMER, N., and WOLFF, H. G.: An examination of the relation between symptoms, disability and serious illness, in two homogenous groups of men and women. *Amer. J. Public Health, 50*:1327-1366, 1960.

95. HINKLE, L. E., JR., KANE, F. D., CHRISTENSON, W. N., and WOLFF, H. G.: Hungarian refugees: Life experiences and features influencing participation in the revolution and subsequent flight. *Amer. J. Psychiat., 116*:16-19, 1959.

96. STUNKARD, A. J., and WOLFF, H. G.: Pathogenesis in human obesity. Function and disorder of a mechanism of satiety. *Psychosom. Med., 20*:17-29, 1958.

97. STUNKARD, A. J., GRACE, W. J., and WOLFF, H. G.: The night eating syndrome. A pattern of food intake among certain obese patients. *Amer. J. Med., 19*:78-86, 1955.

98. HIMWICH, HAROLD E., Ed.: *Alcoholism, Basic Aspects and Treatment.* Washington, American Assoc. Advancement Sc., 1957.

99. *Narcotic Drug Addiction Problems—U.S.P.H.S. Symposium, with Multiple Authorship.* Washington, D.C., U.S. Dept. of Health, Education and Welfare, 1963.

100. SAINSBURY, PETER: *Suicide in London,* Maudsley Monograph, No. 1. New York, Basic Books, 1956.

101. DURKHEIM, EMILE: *Suicide (Translation)* Glencoe, Free Press, 1952.

102. HENDIN, HERBERT H.: *Suicide in Scandinavia. A Psychoanalytic Study of Culture and Character.* New York, Grune and Stratton, 1964.

103. HINKLE, L. E., JR., GITTINGER, J., GOLDBERGER, L., OSTFELD, A., METRAUX, R., RICHTER, P., and WOLFF, H. G.: Studies in human ecology: Factors governing the adaptation of Chinese unable to return to China. In: *Experimental Psychopathology.* New York, Grune and Stratton, 1957, Chap. II, pp. 170-186.

104. HINKLE, L. E., JR., PLUMMER, N., METRAUX, R., RICHTER, P., GITTINGER, J. W., THETFORD, W. N., OSTFELD, A. M., KANE, F. D., GOLDBERGER, LEO, MITCHELL, W. E., LEICHTER, H., PINSKY, R., GOEBEL, D., BROSS, I. D. J., and WOLFF, H. G.: Studies in human ecology. Factors relevant to the occurrence of bodily illness and disturbances in mood, thought and

behavior in three homogeneous population groups. *Amer. J. Psychiat.*, *114*:212-220, 1957.

105. WOLF, STEWART: The implications of social sciences for the future of medicine. Chap. 2 in *Medical Education and Medical Care: Interactions and Prospects*, Report of 8th Teaching Institute, Assn. Am. Med. Colleges, Evanston, 1961.

106. LYND, R. S., and LYND, HELEN M.: *Middletown (1959) and Middletown in Transition (1937)*. New York, Harcourt.

107. WARNER, W. L., and LUNT, P. S.: *The Social Life of a Modern Community*. Yankee City Series, Vol. 1. New Haven, Yale, 1947.

108. WARNER, W. L., and SROLE, L.: *The Social Systems of American Ethnic Groups*. Yankee City Series, Vol. 3. New Haven, Yale, 1945.

109. BENEDICT, RUTH: *Patterns of Culture* (with a new preface by Margaret Mead). Boston, Houghton, 1959 (1934).

110. BENEDICT, RUTH: *The Chrysanthemum and the Sword: Patterns of Japanese Culture*. Boston, Houghton, 1946.

111. GALDSTON, IAGO, Ed.: *Medicine and Anthropology Lectures to the Laity*, No. 21, N. Y. Academy of Medicine. New York, Internat. Univ. Press, 1959.

112. WOLFF, H. G., and HINKLE, L. E., JR.: Human ecology, the central nervous system and disease: Observations relevant to essential hypertension. *Cor Vasa*, *3(1)*:1-32, 1961.

113. PERERA, G.: Hypertensive vascular disease: Description and natural history. *J. Chronic Dis.*, *1*:33, 1955.

114. MOSER, M.: Epidemiology of primary hypertension with particular references to racial susceptibility. In: *Symposium on Hypertension*, Amer. Heart Assn., New York, 1959, p. 72.

115. THOMAS, W. A,. LEE, K. T., and DAOUD, A. S.: Geographic aspects of atherosclerosis. *Ann. Rev. Med.*, *15*:255-72, 1964.

116. PICKERING, SIR GEORGE: *The Nature of Hypertension*. London, Churchill, 1961.

117. SIMONSOM, E., and BROZEK, J.: Russian research on hypertensive disease. *Ann. Intern. Med.*, *50*:129, 1959.

118. HOFFMAN, R.: Blood pressure and subarctic climate in the Soviet Union (Survey of the Russian Literature and Investigations on Delayed Repatriots). Medical Series No. 16, 1958.

119. Symposium on Population Studies in Relation to Chronic Rheumatic Diseases, Rome, 1961. J. H. Kellgren, M. R. Jeffrey, and J. Ball, Eds. UNESCO and WHO, Council of

Internat. Orgs. of Med. Sciences, Oxford, Blackwell Scientific Publications, 1963.

120. HARRIS, L. J.: *Vitamins, in Theory and Practice,* Cambridge Univ. Press, 1955 (4th Ed.).

121. HARRIS, L. J., Ed.: *Garrods Inborn Errors of Metabolism,* London and New York, Oxford Univ. Press, 1955.

122. BLUMBERG, B. S.: Differences in the frequency of disease (Cancer), In: *Different Populations. Ann. Rev. Med., 16*:387-404, 1965.

123. SEGI, M., and KURIHARA, M.: Cancer Mortality for Selected Sites in Twenty-four Countries. Dept. of Public Health, Tohoku University School of Medicine, Japan, 1962.

124. TOOR, M., KATCHALSKY, A., AGMON, J., and ALLALOUF, D.: Atherosis and related factors in immigrants to Israel. *Circulation, 22*:265-79, 1960.

125. BRUNNER, D., and MANELIS, G.: Myocardial infarction among members of communal settlements in Israel. *Lancet, 2*:1049-50, 1960.

126. GROEN, J. J., and LIEBER, E.: Socio-medical aspects of bronchial asthma in Israel. *Israel Med. J., 19*:121-36, 1960.

127. KEYS, ANCEL, KIMURA, NOBORU, KUSUKAWA, AKIRA, BRONTE-STEWART, B., LARSEN, NILS, and KEYS, MARGARET HANEY: Lessons from serum cholesterol studies in Japan, Hawaii and Los Angeles. *Ann. Intern. Med., 48*:83, 1958.

128. HSU, F. L. K.: *The Chinese Hawaii.* Translated by New York Academy of Science, *13*:243, 1951.

129. BEWS, J. W.: *Human Ecology.* London, Oxford, 1935.

Chapter III

ADAPTIVE REACTION PATTERNS

STUDIES OF REACTION PATTERNS involving the various structures of the body are described briefly in this chapter. No attempt is made to offer complete data. Rather, the general nature of reaction patterns is illustrated with reference particularly to studies carried out in the laboratory of Harold Wolff at Cornell-New York Hospital and covering the years 1932-1962. Allusions to the work of others are made for purposes of clarification and extension of the data, but there has been no attempt to provide an exhaustive account of studies relating life stress to bodily disease. The bibliography, however, does include certain references to recent studies, some of which have appeared since Dr. Wolff's death. In addition there are listed at the end of the bibliography several general references not referred to in the text.

THE HEAD

The evolutionary development of man has been characterized by a process of encephalization, or of concentrating more and more the control of bodily function in the most rostral structure. Containing as it does the brain and the end organs of special sense, the head becomes of paramount importance in man's adjustments to his environment. Moreover, as the most prominent and important aspect of the appearance of a man to his fellow man, disorders or disfigurements about the head are likely to arouse more intense anxiety and concern than similar disturbances in other parts of the body. The various structures of the head are dealt with below in relation to symptoms and bodily disease.

HEADACHE

The commonest complaint referable to the head, and perhaps the commonest symptom that confronts physicians, is headache. The most frequently encountered are vascular headaches of the migraine type and muscle contraction (tension) headaches. The latter result from sustained contraction of skeletal muscles about the head and neck which occurs as an individual meets day to day challenges, frustrations and disappointments.

Skeletal muscles comprise the largest bulk of man's bodily tissues and are involved in a great number of his adaptive maneuvers. It is not surprising, therefore, that skeletal muscles participate in a host of adaptive patterns that, when exaggerated or prolonged, become symptomatic. Skeletal muscles are contracted most typically in postures appropriate to alertness and readiness for action. Thus, not only headaches but backaches, periarticular aches, aches in the extremities, and paresthesias may occur in tense, dissatisfied, resentful people because of sustained contraction of skeletal muscles. The headache of muscle tightness occurs in association with cramming for an examination, driving long hours in heavy traffic, and enduring inactivity and boredom. On the other hand such a headache often accompanies a state of sustained alertness, anxiety, tension, and readiness to spring into action, especially if the action fails to come off.

Vascular headaches of the migraine type constitute by far the most troublesome and most incapacitating headaches. They may be of any intensity, from a slight dull ache to a throbbing pain of prostrating severity. The names hemicrania and migraine were applied because these headaches are often confined to one side of the head. In a person having a one-sided vascular headache, the arteries over the temple on the aching side stand out in bold relief, as compared to the other side. Their prominent dilatation and pulsation can be palpated and often seen. Such vascular dilatation and distention causes pain. In most migraine headaches, it is mainly the cranial arteries on the outside of the head which are involved (1, 2) (Fig. 2).

In a long series of experiments, the relation of the intensity of headache to the amplitude of pulsation of the cranial branches

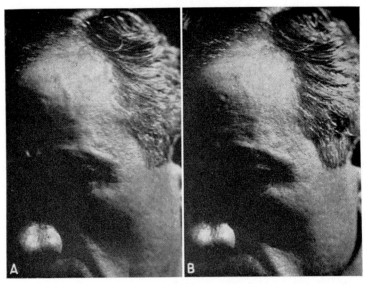

Figure 2. Appearance of the temporal artery before and after termination of migraine headache by ergotamine tartrate. Photograph A was taken while the patient was suffering from a left-sided migraine headache. The temporal arteries stood out clearly. Photograph B was taken under identical conditions twenty minutes later. In the interim, the patient had received ergotamine tartrate (0.4 mg) intravenously, and his headache had been abolished. The temporal vessels were much less prominent.

of the external carotid artery has been demonstrated (2). The intravenous or intramuscular injection of a vasoconstrictor agent, such as ergotamine tartrate, results in a prompt decrease in the amplitude of pulsations of the temporal and occipital arteries which is paralleled by the abolition of the headache (Fig. 3). During a migraine headache attack, sensitivity of the tissues to pressure is predictably increased, and edema accumulates in those areas of the scalp in which headache is being experienced. Specimens of tissue fluid collected from these painful areas during headache were found to contain a substance that could be identified as a polypeptide of the same general type as bradykinin, and after many tests to establish its characteristics, it was named "neurokinin" (3-10). The neurokinin content of tissue fluid collected during headache was eight to thirty-five times as much as that found in control specimens collected in non-headache periods or from persons who have never had headaches. The

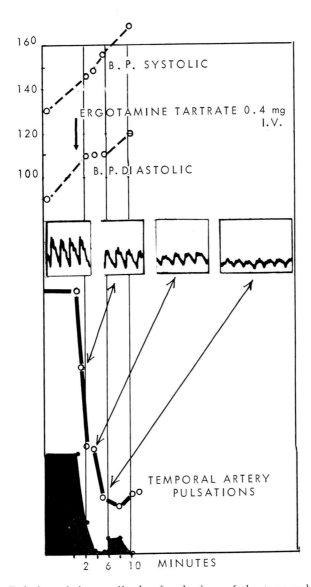

Figure 3. Relation of the amplitude of pulsations of the temporal artery to the intensity of headache (solid black area) after administration of ergotamine tartrate. The sharp decrease in the amplitude of pulsations following injection of ergotamine closely paralleled the rapid decrease in intensity of the headache. Representative sections of the photographic record are inserted.

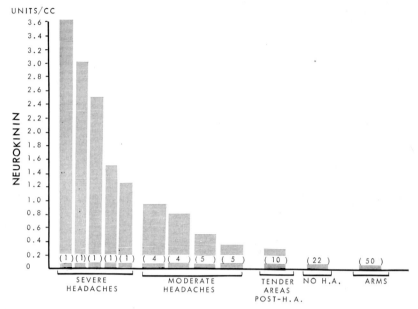

Figure 4. Results of bioassay of subcutaneous perfusates grouped according to the intensity of pain. "Neurokinin" activity was assayed on a strip of rat duodenum. Amounts recovered from the scalp are compared with a control area, the subcutaneous tissue of the forearm (right hand column).

quantity of neurokinin activity in the specimens recovered was closely related to the intensity of the headache (Fig 4). The increased content of this polypeptide found locally can account for many of the features of vascular headache of the migraine type. Neurokinin is also released into the skin of man elsewhere than the head during neuronal excitation, such as antidromic dorsal root stimulation and during axon reflex flare. A powerful vasodilator, neurokinin, when injected into the skin of man, induced pain and reddening, lowered pain thresholds, and increased capillary permeability. These findings suggest that neurokinin serves in local vasomotor control for the central nervous system.

Although the pain of headache is attributable to arterial dilatation, the vascular headache syndrome may begin with vasoconstriction involving intracranial as well as extracranial arteries, even affecting the blood supply of the cerebral cortex or the retina. Thus alarming transitory weakness, paresthesias, scotomata, and even partial blindness may occur (11). The frequent oc-

currence of an initial pallor of the face suggests that vasoconstriction always occurs as the initial phase of a migraine attack,
but since it doesn't ordinarily involve important structures such
as cortex or retina, it may go unnoticed. Whether or not the
subsequent vasodilator phase represents an over-reaction to the
threat to the brain of vasoconstriction cannot be stated on the
basis of current evidence, but it is significant that the branches of
the external and internal carotid arteries have a common innervation which could lead to a simultaneous release of vasodilator
and pain threshold lowering substances both intracranially and
extracranially.

VASOMOTOR INSTABILITY AND VASCULAR HEADACHE

A striking characteristic of those who suffer periodically
from vascular headache is that their extracranial arterial pulsations describe a wider excursion, even in headache free periods,
than do those of nonheadache-prone individuals. The greatest
variability in cranial artery behavior was observed in the days

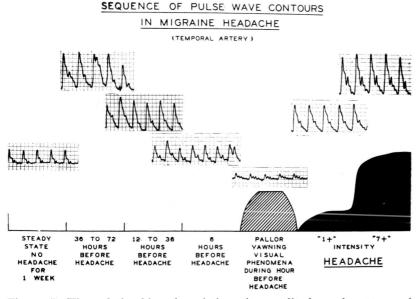

Figure 5. The relationship of variations in amplitude and pattern of
pulsation of a branch of the superficial temporal artery in man to the
phenomena of vascular headache.

immediately preceding a migraine attack. Other vascular beds, including the smaller vessels of the conjunctivae and the nasal mucosae and those concerned with the regulation of arterial pressure and fluid balance have also been found to display a noteworthy lability of behavior in those with vascular headache (12, 13) (Fig. 5).

Pfeiffer and Kunkle (14) demonstrated variation in the responsiveness of cranial vessels to histamine. Smaller amounts of this agent initiated dilatation during periods when the subject was under stress from interpersonal and cultural pressures than during periods of tranquility. Also, it was found that the minute conjunctival vessels exhibited increased sensitiveness to the vasoconstrictor effect of nor-epinephrine in the pre-headache period; and diminished sensitivity during the phase of dilatation and pain. These observations lend support to the concept that the cranial vasomotor apparatus of patients with vascular headache is more labile than is that of those not subject to headache.

MODIFICATION OF VASCULAR REACTIVITY

Recently, the possibility of shedding further light on the pathophysiology of vascular headache of the migraine type was suggested by the reports of a number of investigators that 1-methyl-D-lysergic acid butanolamide bimaleate, while lacking the capacity to terminate an existing headache, is often effective in reducing the number and severity of headache attacks when adequate blood levels are maintained. Although the agent does not by itself induce vasoconstriction, it does enhance the vasoconstrictor action of norepinephrine (13).

Studies with the agent (1-methyl-D-lysergic acid butanolamide bimaleate*) have shown that after several days of administration it is effective in dampening a variety of vascular reactions in animals and humans. These include an anti-inflammatory reaction and the mitigation of pressor responses to cold or breath holding (13). The effects of the agent, as observed in a variety of acute and chronic experiments indicate an inhibitory action on central vasoconstrictor reflexes, and a peripheral action of enhancing vasoconstriction induced by catecholamines. It was

*UML-491, Sandoz ® Sansert.

observed that the modulating effects of the agent on vasomotor responses were most marked in those patients who experienced the most striking interruption of their headaches (15-18).

DAMPING EFFECT OF UML-491 ON BLOOD VESSEL RESPONSIVENESS

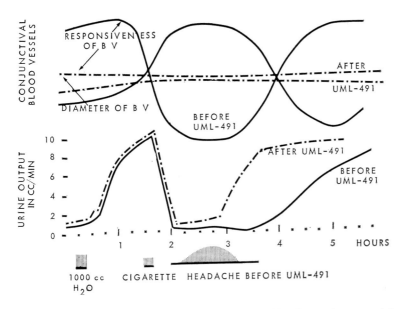

Figure 6. The damping effect of UML-491 on blood vessel responsivity in overhydrated subjects in whom oliguria is induced, the conjunctival blood vessels become dilated and the response of these vessels to serial dilutions of norepinephrine is diminished (from about 1:200.000 to about 1:50.000). During the spontaneous diuresis which follows induced oliguria, the dilated conjunctival blood vessels become slightly constricted, and the response of these vessels to serial dilutions of norepinephrine is returned to the preoliguria status. These changes in vascular diameter and responsivity to vasoconstrictor agents were related to the duration and degree of the induced oliguria and subsequent diuresis, being more profound in those patients in whom the fluid shifts were most striking. The prior administration of UML-491 reduced the magnitude of these vascular responses, especially during oliguria.

These data suggest that in the prophylaxis of vascular headache of the migraine type the magnitude of cranial vascular responsivity is reduced, thereby preventing the crises of vaso-constriction and vasodilatation that characterize the migraine attack. These observations further support the thesis that migraine is the symptomatic manifestation of recurrent heightened reactivity of cranial blood vessels.

PERSONALITY AND HEREDITY IN MIGRAINE

Migraine headaches are linked to activity of the central nervous system since they most often occur during or after a long period of alertness, with obsessive striving to continue difficult tasks and maintain schedules, with extraordinary effort and excessive output of energy, and usually with accompanying feelings of anger and resentment (1-10).

In a study of their personality profiles, scores of subjects suffering from these vascular headaches revealed their dominant features, attitudes, and reactions to be feelings of insecurity and tension manifested as inflexibility, conscientiousness, meticulousness, perfectionism and resentment (19). The elaboration of a pattern of inflexibility and perfectionism for dealing with feelings of insecurity begins early in childhood. The individual with migraine aims to gain approval by doing more than and better than his fellows through "application" and "hard work," and to gain security by holding to a stable environment and a given system of excellent performance, even at a high cost of energy. This pattern brings the individual increasing responsibility and admiration with but little love, and greater and greater resentment at the pace he feels obliged to maintain. Then the tension associated with repeated frustration, sustained resentment and anxiety is often followed by prostrating fatigue and becomes the setting in which the migraine attack occurs (19).

Systematic study of the family trees of 119 patients with migraine revealed highly significant evidence of the hereditary character of the trait. Perhaps such individuals have a predisposition and psychobiologic equipment which makes them prone to sustained and pernicious emotional states and to labile regulatory mechanisms of the cranial vasculature (18).

In any case, migraine headaches occur when hereditarily susceptible persons attempt to control feelings of anxiety and resentment by means of organized and intense activity. It is thus a cranial vascular consequence of a way of life. So predictable is this behavior pattern in migraine patients that the interested physician can demonstrate it in nearly every subject he examines.

A striking demonstration of the effects of attitudes was made by Marcussen, who was able to precipitate headache predictably in certain patients by stress-inducing interviews in which topics of personal importance were discussed in such a way that the patients developed intense feelings of resentment and guilt (20). Under these circumstances, discussions lasting approximately one hour were followed by typical migraine headaches which could be terminated by ergotamine tartrate

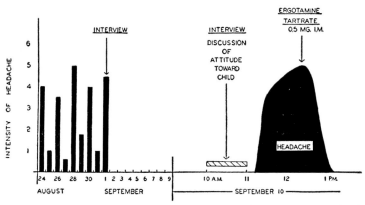

Figure 7. Precipitation of a migraine headache in a woman following a discussion of her feelings of guilt and resentment toward her child.

administered intramuscularly. Subsequent encouragement of these patients to recognize their attitudes as the reason for their angry reactions and helping them to modify their attitudes resulted in diminution of both the frequency and intensity of headache attacks (Fig. 7).

At the time of his death, Harold Wolff was still exploring the biologic significance of vascular headache of the migraine type. He had shown the biphasic vascular reaction, vasoconstriction and vasodilatation, and he had demonstrated that both intracranial and extracranial structures were involved in the reaction pattern. Finally, and perhaps most important, he had discovered neurokinin, the neurohumor elaborated in the tissues as a result of excitation in the central nervous system (1, 5-8). Had he lived, his final hypothesis that the disordered vaso-activity reflected an adaptive response to a threat to the integrity of the brain itself would have been put to further test.

THE EYES

In contrast to other mammals who depend primarily on ears, nose and vibrissae for orientation, man's eyes are pre-dominant in relating him to his environment. The highly specialized and delicate mechanisms of the eye offer many oppor-tunities for disorder and disease, among them disturbances in the coordination of extra- and intra-ocular muscles.

Sours and Erdbrink (21) describe the phenomenology of ciliary muscle spasm leading to false myopia in a series of nineteen aviators. These patients showed evidence of depression, fear and conflicts involving guilt. When removed from their stressful circumstances, i.e., when excused from flying, the visual symptoms cleared.

Dachryocystitis is considered by ophthalmologists to be frequently attributable to difficulties in emotional adjustment and related to excessive lacrimation although the manifestations of inflammation of the tear glands have not been subjected to careful experimental study (22). In the eye itself, the retina has been found to participate in adaptive reactions during stress, most typically as a result of arterial constriction during the prodrome of an attack of migraine headache, as described in Section I. Long lasting scotomata have also been observed and sometimes total blindness, as part of a hysterical reaction.

Wolf and Ripley (23) found optic atrophy and paracentral scotomata widespread among American, British, and Dutch prisoners of war of the Japanese. In some subjects, scotomata were consistently demonstrated without pallor of the discs. In these subjects, the scotomata were dispelled after an intravenously administered hypnotic amobarbital sodium, and strong reassur-ance.

One of the most intriguing ocular lesions found to be associated with protective adaptive reactions was phlyctenular keratitis (24). In a setting of repeated conflicts with his mother, a sullen rebellious youth displayed attacks of intense engorgement of corneal vessels associated with lachrymation, photophobia, nasal obstruction and rhinorrhea. He had developed a full-blown phlyctenular keratitis by the time he was first seen in the clinic. His typical attacks were induced repeatedly by discussion of his relations with his mother while his corneal vessels were under observation through a slit lamp. As his relationship with his physician became firm and constructive, and as he began to understand his problems, spontaneous attacks occurred less frequently, and finally largely subsided. At this time, a bilateral corneal transplant was successfully performed, and with continued close association with his physician, further attacks of corneal hyperemia were kept at a minimum.

Certain forms of glaucoma, one of the most menacing of eye diseases, were recognized as greatly influenced by life adjustment early in the present century by the ophthalmologist Laqueur (25), himself a victim of the disease. Ripley and Wolff (26), studying eighteen patients with varying degrees of glaucoma, were able readily to correlate intraocular pressure with life situation and emotional reaction. It was also possible in these and in certain healthy subjects to induce a rise in intraocular tension by a discussion with the subject of his significant personal conflicts.

It would appear, therefore, that the eyes participate in man's adjustments to his surroundings to a degree comparable to their importance in adaptation. In each instance, the pathological feature appears to represent an exaggeration in degree, or duration, or both of a normal function. Some of the mechanisms which may be involved in such excessive and seemingly inappropriate behavior will be discussed in Chapter IV.

THE AIRWAYS

The nose, the bronchi and the lungs carry on a continuous exchange between man and his environment and may become involved in protective adaptive reactions of various sorts (27).

A. The Nose

Smell, a sensation so basic to the adjustment of a great many vertebrates and especially mammals, seems almost vestigial in man. The olfactory cortex and the limbic system which serve to integrate information from olfactory structures in the lower animals appear to be taken up with the formulation and expression of emotions in man in response to a wide variety of afferent impulses in addition to smell. Nevertheless, certain odors for man are powerfully symbolic of past experiences and feeling states. Certain structural diseases of the brain are associated with hallucinations of smell. Little information, however, is available on disorders of smell function as part of an adaptive process.

"Air conditioning," for man probably the most important function of the nose, is the process of warming and moistening inspired air and filtering it to some degree so that it is in a suitable state to encounter the delicate alveolar surfaces of the lungs. When inspired air is contaminated by noxious substances such as smoke, or the fumes of certain chemicals the nose is capable of affording a degree of protection through swelling of the turbinates and an increased flow of mucus. Such a reaction, which has been called the bodily response of "shutting out and washing away" when extreme, results in complete occlusion of the nares so that whatever breathing occurs takes place via the relatively unprotected throat.

The reaction of "shutting out and washing away" is characteristic of the syndrome, vasomotor rhinitis. It involves hyperemia of the conjunctivae and lacrimation and was aroused experimentally by a series of noxious stimuli, first tangible and directed against the airways, then against the person and finally delivered as symbols.

Effects of Noxious Stimuli

In experimental sessions, after establishing a base line for nasal function, subjects were exposed to a series of graded threats beginning with those directed specifically at the nasorespiratory passages.

Irritant Fumes

Inhalation for one minute of ammonium carbonate fumes provoked the expected reaction; namely, after inhalation, sudden hyperemia and swelling of the nasal structures with hypersecretion and obstruction. Associated with these nasal changes there occurred lacrimation and spasm of the eyelids, as well as strenuous coughing (Fig. 8).

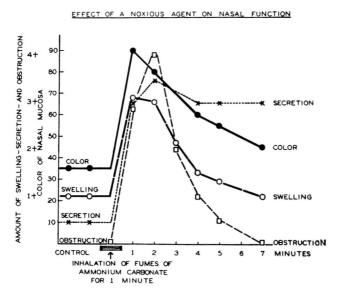

Figure 8. Hyperemia with swelling of the nasal mucous membranes, hypersecretion and obstruction of the airways following inhalation of irritant fumes.

This appeared to be a protective reaction on the part of the organism, an effort at shutting out, washing away, neutralizing, and ejecting the offending substance.

Pollen

Another type of assault against the person arises from the inhalation of pollens to which he may be sensitive. Accordingly, a subject was studied in an attack of hay fever. Prior to the attack, the septum and turbinates were comparatively pale and appeared normal. Immediately upon beginning to cut flowers in his garden,

however, the subject began to weep and sneeze. His membranes
had become hyperemic, wet, and swollen (Fig. 9).

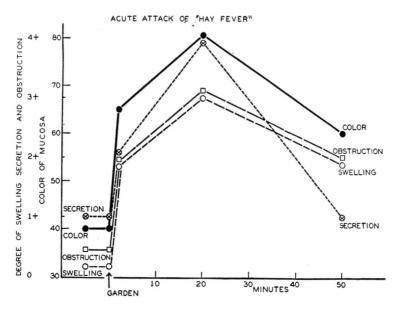

Figure 9. Hyperemia and swelling of the nasal mucosae, hypersecretion and
obstruction of the airways during an abortive attack of "hay fever," following
exposure to pollens.

This particular attack was an abortive one, but it was frequently observed that when the swelling of the membranes was
sustained, the hyperemia subsided, leaving the membranes pale
but swollen, wet and edematous. This pale, swollen state is the
usual appearance of the nose of the hay fever sufferer when he
comes to the doctor's office for treatment. It would appear, however, that as in the case of inhalation of irritating fumes, the
hyperemia comes first, thus providing another instance in which
the protective bodily reaction of shutting out and washing away
may be invoked.

Pain

The next step was to inflict upon the experimental subject a
nonspecific threat, not directed at his respiratory passages. Accord-

ingly, the head was constricted in a tight-fitting steel crown which gave rise to an intense headache. This was a highly unpleasant experience, associated with feelings of apprehension on the part of the subject, and development of the same protective reaction as that described above for more specific threats to the nose (Fig. 10).

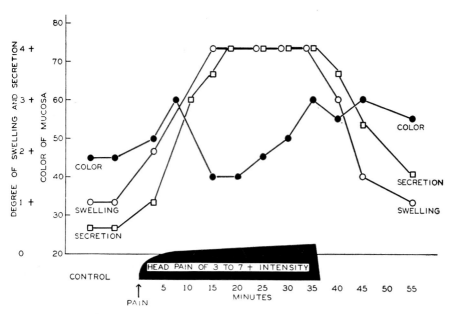

CHANGES IN NASAL FUNCTION DURING INDUCED HEAD PAIN

Figure 10. Hyperemia, hypersecretion and obstruction in the nose during induced headache- a nasal reaction to a non-specific threat.

Word Symbols

The final aim was to learn whether or not symbolic threats which did not involve the application of physical trauma would induce such a protective pattern with nasal changes.

A sufferer from chronic rhinitis whose nasal structures at the time of observation were normal was forcibly reminded that he was caught in the toils of an unfavorable marriage, that his wife was using him for a meal ticket and giving him nothing in return. He promptly began to display the evidences of nasal hyperfunc-

tioning noted above and there was an almost complete obstruction
to breathing. He described himself as being on the verge of tears
although weeping did not occur. After the discussion was ended,
the subject was reassured and diverted and after another hour the
nasal functions had returned toward normal (Fig. 11).

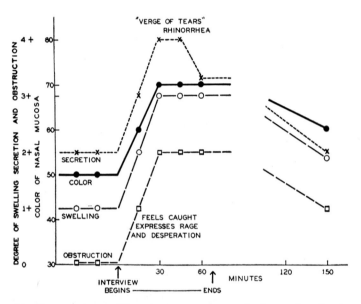

Figure 11. Hyperemia, swelling, hypersecretion and obstruction in the nose
experimentally induced during an interview in which the subject experienced
feelings of rage and desperation.

The association of nasal hyperfunction with weeping was frequently observed. The fact that the tears pass into the nose
through the nasolacrimal duct may be of some significance with
regard to the nasal changes which accompany weeping, but it
seems unlikely that the chemical composition of tears is sufficiently irritating to produce hyperemia and swelling, and indeed
the changes in the nose often occurred without actual lacrimation.
Lacrimation, like nasal hypersecretion, serves to wash away par-
ticles and to dilute noxious agents. The origin of nasal hyperfunction may be related in some way to weeping in childhood and
occur as part of a conditional response. The individual may continue to use the physiologic pattern effective against noxae in the
air to gain sympathy, support and protection for himself against

many other threats from a hostile environment. As the individual grows older, he may perpetuate the inappropriate weeping pattern as a way of life, despite the fact that it becomes progressively less effective as protection against symbolic threats and assaults. Perhaps this concept will answer Tennyson's query, "Tears, idle tears, I know not what they mean" (28). The complete weeping pattern, involving both the eyes and the nose, often persists in females into adult life. In adult males, however, the impact of cultural conditioning fragments the pattern, and frank weeping is seldom manifest, although hyperfunction in the nose may be readily evoked. (See Chapter IV.)

Structural Tissue Changes and Cellular Reactions

Biopsy of Turbinates

In an attempt to explore the characteristics of the nasal mem-

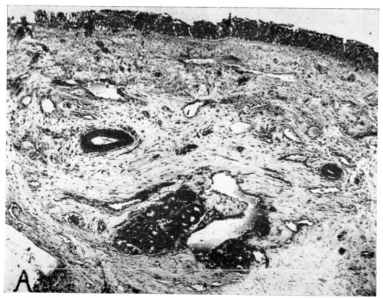

Figure 12. Biopsies from the nasal mucous membrane of a 36-year-old man with chronic vasomotor rhinitis before and after interview engendering nasal hyperfunction and conflict. (a) Biopsy of the left lower turbinate obtained before interview when nasal function was within average limits. Section shows low grade chronic inflammation, relatively undilated vascular and lymphatic channels and compact, quiescent mucous glands. There is no edema of the stroma.

branes during hyperfunction, a biopsy was made from the inferior
turbinate of a sufferer from chronic rhinitis, first on one side during a control period of rest and relaxation when the membranes
were in an average state of activity, and again, from the opposite
turbinate, at the height of a frustrating interview when the patient
was on the verge of tears. Both biopsies were made with the same
technique and the same topical cocaine anesthesia. The first section showed an essentially normal mucosal structure with moderate round-cell infiltration. The second revealed the mucous glands
to be filled with secretion and the vascular and lymphatic channels
to be prominent and dilated. In addition, there was interstitial
edema (Fig. 12a & b).

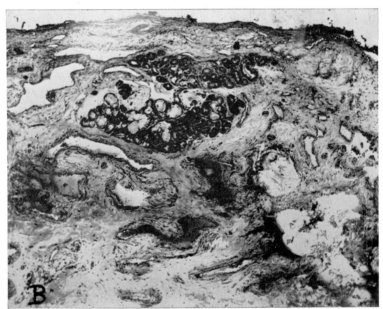

(b) Biopsy of the right lower turbinate obtained one hour later, at the
point of maximal nasal hyperfunction accompanying intense conflict and
"verge of tears." Section shows prominent, dilated vascular and lymphatic
channels, active mucous glands filled with secretion. Lighter value of the
stroma indicates edema. (Magnification x200, Masson's Trichrome Stain.)

Nasal secretions of subjects with rhinitis were collected and
stained by an appropriately standardized technique before, during,

and after the discussion of significant conflicts. At the same time, white blood cell counts were made on the peripheral blood. It was found that nasal hyperfunction in association with such induced stress was accompanied by a marked eosinophila in the secretions and in the peripheral blood as well. The reaction is illustrated in Fig. 13. In this subject, as well as in others, an eosinophilic reaction associated with stress was accompanied by a purulent response characterized by the presence of polymorphonuclear leucocytes in the nasal secretions.

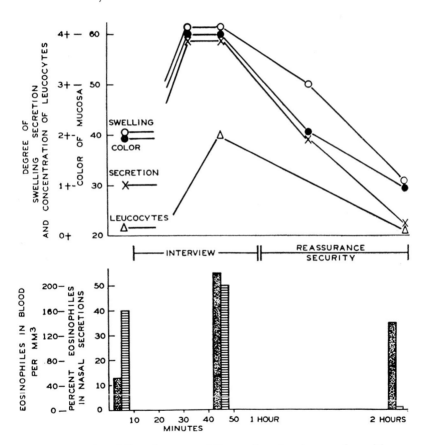

Figure 13. Eosinophil and neutrophil reaction in the nasal cavities, accompanying feelings of resentment, frustration, humiliation and guilt. (Stippled bars represent number of eosinophils in circulating blood.)

Tissue Fragility and Pain Threshold

Other evidence of "organic" tissue changes in the nose in response to symbolic threats to the integrity or welfare of the organism were found to be increased fragility of the membranes and lowered pain threshold accompanying sustained nasal hyperfunction. Ordinarily, when the membranes were in their average state, minor traumata with the nasal speculum were neither significantly painful nor productive of bleeding. Under circumstances of sustained hyperemia, however, the merest contact of speculum with turbinate was intensely painful and usually resulted in erosion and bleeding.

The Relative Importance of Pollen and Life Situations In Inducing Nasal Hyperfunctions and Eosinophilia

Since eosinophilia, widely considered pathognomonic of allergy, was observed as a part of the bodily reaction to induced stress (see Fig. 14), it became especially interesting to compare this eosinophilic reaction with that induced by pollens. Accord-

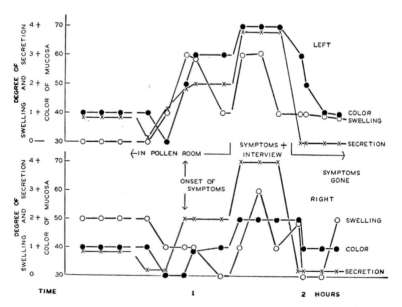

Figure 14. Combined effect of troublesome life situation and pollen on nasal function response.

ingly, two groups of subjects, including those with strictly seasonal ragweed hay fever, those with nonseasonal vasomotor rhinitis but with and without skin sensitivity to ragweed, were selected and studied by the above methods. In addition, they were exposed to measured amounts of mixed ragweed pollen circulating in the air of a special pollen room without their being aware of it. These experiments were performed both in and out of ragweed hay fever season.

Of special interest was an experiment on the twenty-one-year-old girl of Figure 14 who had had strictly seasonal ragweed hay fever. The steel band was adjusted to her head so as to induce headache, an experience to which she submitted, but vigorously resented. She couldn't have been allergically sensitized to this experience since she had never had it before. Nevertheless, eosinophiles again appeared in her nasal secretions in significant numbers, just as they had at the time of the discussion of significant personal conflicts during ragweed season, but when her nasal membranes were fairly normal eosinophiles both in the nasal secretions and in the blood were at a low level.

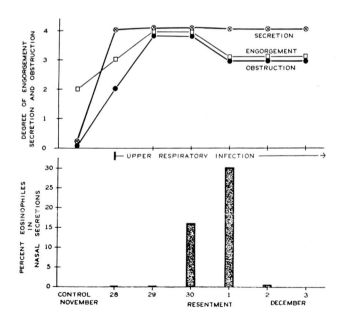

Figure 15. Eosinophilia induced during a head cold at a time of resentment.

Generally speaking, with or without skin sensitivity, those subjects who did not have strictly seasonal hay fever failed to react to the inhalation of mixed ragweed pollen unless their nasal membranes were already somewhat hyperemic from one cause or another (29). However, when there was pre-existing nasal hyperfunction from whatever cause, not only those subjects, but non-hay fever sufferers as well, often reacted to the pollen room experience with marked hyperfunction, weeping, and sneezing. Such typical hay fever attacks were often induced when pollen inhalation was undertaken during spontaneously occurring difficult life situations productive of conflict. Furthermore, it was possible during pollen inhalation in the absence of nasal hyperfunction to induce an attack of frank hay fever by a discussion of significant personal problems and to induce subsidence of the attack by reassurance while the pollen was still being inhaled.

One subject (Fig. 15) had no ragweed sensitivity and never had symptoms of rhinitis except for occasional head colds. At such times, however, it was possible by adding further insult, either locally to her membrane or generally to her pride, to induce an intensification of her symptoms, with eosinophilia.

The Contrast of Hyperfunction and Hypofunction

The attitudes of individuals with vasomotor rhinitis and asthma are remarkably similar to the "shutting out-washing away" reaction that is so descriptive of the behavior of their nasal mucous membranes and bronchi in response to chemical and symbolic assaults. These attitudes express a desire for non-participation and have been studied in a large group of patients, notably by Grace and Graham (30, 31).

Cannon (32), years ago, described a contrasting respiratory reaction occurring in emotionally significant circumstances, namely, shrinkage of the mucosa with resulting enlargement of the airways. He interpreted this as a preparation for flight or fight and saw it as a useful bodily adjustment to allow a greater access of oxygen to the lungs.

It was possible to confirm Cannon's findings in human beings, inducing pallor of the nasal mucosa and increased breathing space, under overwhelming circumstances of fright or dejection. For example, a physician who usually reacted to situational threats with blocking off of nasal passages—the shutting out and washing away pattern—on one occasion when his pregnant wife had a suddent hemoptysis, was terrified, and responded with shrinkage, pallor and dryness of the nasal mucosae (27).

B. The Bronchi and Bronchial Secretions

The mucous membrane of the nose and pharynx is continuous with that of the bronchi and is histologically closely similar. Hence, it is not surprising that the bronchi themselves often participate in reaction patterns involving the nose. The mucosal engorgement and narrowing of the bronchial channels as well as the excess of mucous secretion characteristic of asthmatic attacks resembles closely the hyperfunctioning state of the nose already described.

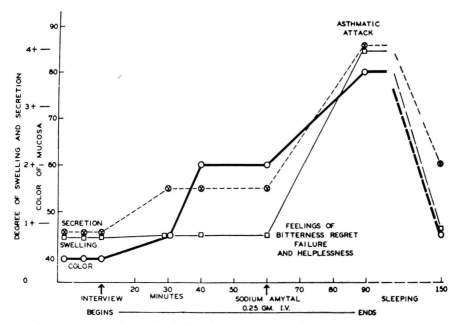

Figure 16. Experimentally induced hyperemia, swelling, hypersecretion and obstruction in the nose associated with narrowing of the bronchial tubes during a discussion of topics provoking feelings of bitterness, regret, failure and helplessness. The subject experienced an "asthmatic attack."

Two groups of patients, those with cutaneous sensitivity to pollens, and those free of evidence of such sensitivity were studied over relatively long periods of time in relation to their life experience. Attacks of asthma often coincide with periods of situational conflict among both the "sensitive" and "non-sensitive" subjects. Experiments carried out in the pollen room referred to above (29) yielded findings similar to those reported for the nose. In addition it was possible to induce typical evidences of acute asthma, including dyspnoea, wheezing and coughing productive of tenacious mucoid sputum in suitably susceptible subjects by initiating a discussion of emotionally troublesome topics (27). For example, a thirty-six-year-old housewife had been subject to typical frequently recurring asthmatic attacks, over the past eight years. Her parents were strict, religiously observant, orthodox Jews, born in Russia. Her father, who had been a Rabbi, took an inordinate pride in his daughter's precocious attainments in school and was at the same time over-restrictive. At age seventeen, the girl had a frustrating love affair with a young lawyer who unwittingly humiliated her because he considered her "too young" for his amorous advances. In rebellion, the patient married secretly a Roman Catholic Merchant sailor. The latter proved to be unambitious and a poor provider. The patient was determined to vindicate her position by earning enough to educate their children. Vasomotor rhinitis began when the oldest child was discovered to have diabetes, thus requiring her to give up her job and stay at home to prepare a special diet. The following year the first of her asthmatic attacks appeared at the time her second child also manifested symptoms suggestive of diabetes. On several occasions, typical attacks of asthma were induced in this patient by the technique of the "Stress Interview" described in Chapter II. Figure 16 illustrates one such experiment. The nasal structures were kept under observation through a suitable speculum and auscultation of her chest was repeatedly carried out. During the initial control period, the nasal membranes were of normal appearance and the chest was clear. As a discussion of the discovery of diabetes in her oldest child was undertaken, the nasal mucosae became swollen, wet and hyperemic. At the same time, wheezing and coughing began. Thirty minutes later she was given intravenously 0.25 gm sodium amytal. She became relaxed, smiled, and her asthma subsided.

The subject of the Jewish lawyer she had loved was introduced, together with a consideration of her reasons for throwing away opportunities for marital happiness, economic security, productive offspring and favor with her family. She indicated that she felt caught in a trap. Her voice became weak and wheezing and coughing began again, associated with a marked increase in nasal hyperaemia, secretion and swelling. Uutimately, the discussion was dropped and the patient slept. On awakening, there was still slight wheezing and occasional cough but the nasal mucosal swelling had largely subsided.

In addition to the changes in the bronchial mucosa and musculature characteristic of the asthmatic attack, there appears to be an element involving skeletal muscles, the intercostal musculature and the diaphragm. Groen (33) has shown that an asthmatic attack can be simulated voluntarily by sudden forceful expiratory efforts. In experimental studies of patients subject to asthmatic attacks, he was able to induce the full picture of asthma during stressful interviews.

Chronic manifestations of disease of the bronchi usually involve the hypersecretion of mucus. Stevenson (34) showed in a subject with bronchiectasis that the quantity of mucus produced varied strikingly with the subject's prevailing state of emotional adjustment. When an excess of mucus interferes with bronchial drainage, there is little doubt that the hazard of pulmonary infection is increased.

C. Hyperventilation

Other reaction patterns involving respiratory structures include the well known hyperventilation syndrome with its metabolic sequellae which occurs so characteristically under circumstances of acute and often repressed anxiety.

A thirty-four-year-old woman, whose husband was in the Army overseas, complained of attacks of nocturnal dyspnea (35). She was interviewed while she lay quietly on her bed. Records of her respiration had been taken before and after a standard two-step exercise and in her relaxed state before the interview. During the interview, she complained of her isolation and loneliness because of her husband's absence. She described her perfectionistic employer, his inordinate demands, and her difficult work conditions which made "perfect work" impossible. Her employer's disapproval of her performance deeply hurt and enraged the patient, herself a perfectionist also. Before her husband's departure, she was able at the end of a day to voice her anger and regain her personal dignity through her husband's sympathy and support. Being an aloof person, she had no one to confide in during his absence. Although she expressed no anger, inwardly she was boiling with rage. She even had murderous dreams. Respiratory studies demonstrated that following a discussion of her troubles there was a doubling of the minute ventilation as the utilization coefficient decreased by half, without significant alteration in oxygen consumption. This effect was similar to that observed during strenuous exercise, although the patient had not moved from her bed.

D. Diaphragmatic Spasm

Sudden diaphragmatic spasm is a frequent cause of dyspnea and chest pain. Similar to the familiar "stitch in the side" of runners, it has been observed and induced experimentally in susceptible individuals during situations of strong emotional conflict and may easily be confused with the manifestations of myocardial infarction (36).

The large number of neural connections, afferent and efferent, between the respiratory apparatus and the various levels of central nervous integration attests not only to the obvious importance of breathing mechanisms but also to the potential for acute and chronic disturbances thereof (37, 38).

E. Infections

Infection involving the airways, especially the common cold and respiratory "flu" together with "intestinal flu" are among the most important causes of discomfort and disability for man (27, 39). To investigate the possibility suggested by other work on dif-

ferences in the prevalence of illness in two groups of young men
(40, 41) that some manifest upper respiratory infections might
occur in relation to stressful life experiences, twenty-four women
were selected from an industrial population of 18,000 and studied
by Hinkle and Christenson (42). They were of comparable age,
race, social class and family structure. Careful records were kept
of their health, work and their situation in the home and community. Also, the nasal mucosae were periodically examined and
photographed and serological, bacterial, and virus studies were
made. Fifty episodes of transitory incapacitating illness occurred
among the twenty-four women during a six-month period of intensive study. The episodes were manifested by one or more of the
following: fever, malaise, aching, cough, nausea and diarrhea. All
but seven of the episodes were preceded by a period of nasal
stuffiness associated with hyperemia, engorgement and hypersecretion of the nasal mucosae.

The women with chronic nasal hyperfunction, and those who
exhibited more frequent, more prolonged and more pronounced
upper respiratory reactions had a much greater likelihood of
becoming ill than could be explained on the assumption of equal
risk, a greater likelihood of exhibiting "typically infectious" upper
respiratory illnesses and a much greater likelihood of being disabled by these illnesses.

From the serologic data, several of the women could be said
to have been infected by the virus of "Asian" flu. The manifestations of illness, however—malaise, fever, respiratory and gastrointestinal symptoms—did not correlate closely with the serologic
evidence of infection. On the other hand, the "flu-like" syndromes
correlated strikingly with periods of more or less intense emotional turmoil. Furthermore, the illnesses occurred most frequently in those women whose life adjustment was most
precarious.

Mouth, Saliva and Teeth

The structures of the mouth are involved in a great many
interactions of a human being with his environment. It is not
surprising, therefore, that they respond to circumstances of important symbolic significance. The suppression of saliva, associated

with fear and guilt has been recognized since ancient times when in China a deficiency of saliva was sought among those suspected of crimes by forcing them to chew rice.

Less obvious, but perhaps occurring as frequently in emotionally charged situations, is an increase in salivary secretion. Bogdonoff *et al.*, collected saliva directly from Stenson's duct before and during tooth drilling as their subjects sat in the dentist's chair (43). The individuals were independently evaluated with respect to their personality structure and way of life, and, without knowledge of the salivary data, were classified as preponderantly assertive or on the whole as passive. There was a highly significant correlation between these evaluations and the salivary data. The assertive group secreted increased amounts of saliva during the drilling procedure, while the salivary flow of the passive subjects decreased sharply and assumed a sticky, ropey quality associated with the sudden manifestation of halitosis (44). Such changes were brought on repeatedly in susceptible individuals during "stress interviews."

Dentists have noted the association of dental caries with periods of difficult life adjustment, but there is scanty information as to the mechanisms that may be involved. Spongy gums, on the other hand, and even gingivitis and pyorrhea may be related to vascular changes in the gingiva which accompany adaptive reactions to challenges in day to day life.

Vincents angina, aphthous ulcers and herpes simplex, while clearly associated with infectious agents, nevertheless have been frequently noted to occur during periods of adverse life adjustment and stress evoking circumstances.

The Esophagus

The function of the esophagus is to expedite the passage of swallowed food into the stomach by nicely regulated peristaltic contractions. The propulsive rhythm may be disturbed by a variety of circumstances and in certain disease processes. The studies of Wolf and Almy (45) showed that the motor function of the esophagus is subject to influence by the highest integrative levels of the central nervous system in response to troublesome life situations. Dysrhythmic motor activity, and delay in esophageal empty-ing were identified in several healthy subjects in whom intense headache was induced with the steel head band described earlier under "Airways," and also in students at times of particularly difficult academic examinations. In patients with clinical cardio-spasm, delay in esophageal emptying was induced during "stress interviews" and dispelled by offering strong reassurance.

The Stomach

Investigation of gastric function in man was greatly facilitated by an opportunity to study an individual, Tom, with a large per-manent gastric fistula (46, 47). Tom underwent a surgical gas-trostomy at the age of nine because of an esophageal stricture which resulted from accidentally swallowing scalding hot clam chowder. He was studied more or less intensively from 1941 until his death in 1958.

Two distinct patterns of reaction involving the stomach were identified: the first was characterized by hyperemia and engorge-ment of the mucosa, increased secretion of HCl, and enhanced motor activity, with consequent rapid gastric emptying; the sec-ond was characterized by pallor of the mucosa and depressed activ-ity as regards HCl secretion and motility.

Gastric Hyperfunction

Increased gastric secretion and motor activity occur period-ically at meal times but were also evoked by situations engendering conscious or unconscious anxiety, resentment and hostility (Fig. 17). Transitory gastric hyperfunction was often observed in healthy subjects during brief periods of emotional conflict. Sus-tained changes of this type occurred in situations of chronic conflict, and were accompanied by the typical hunger pains of peptic ulcer, even when no ulcer was present (Fig. 18). Hy-peremia and engorgement of the gastric mucosa when sustained was found to be associated with a lowered pain threshold so that ordinarily non-noxious stimuli such as forceful contractions of the stomach, induced pain. Sustained gastric hyperfunction was

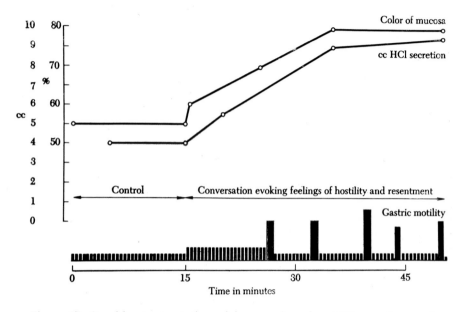

Figure 17. Graphic representation of increase in color, HCl secretion, and motor activity during anxiety characterized by hostility and resentment (observed in subject "Tom" with a gastric fistula) in connection with being unjustly accused of irresponsibility and ineffectiveness.

also accompanied by increased fragility of the mucous membrane to the extent that relatively minor traumata induced erosion and bleeding. Indeed, erosions sometimes appeared spontaneously in the engorged mucosa of the stomach, resulting presumably from the extra vigorous movements of the stomach wall. One such erosion kept in more or less continuous contact with acid gastric juice for a period of three days actually ulcerated, displaying a sharply defined hemorrhagic border and a granulating base, shown in Figure 19.

It is well established that the stomach of the patient with duodenal ulcer is an hyperfunctioning one. Indeed, frequent insult to the duodenal mucosa from the hypersecreting and hypermotile stomach is widely accepted as the pathogenic mechanism of duodenal ulcer. It is therefore particularly significant that studies of patients with duodenal ulcer have revealed them

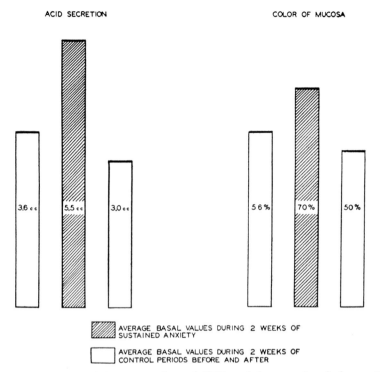

ACID SECRETION   COLOR OF MUCOSA

3,6 cc   5,5 cc   3,0 cc   56%   70%   50%

AVERAGE BASAL VALUES DURING 2 WEEKS OF
SUSTAINED ANXIETY

AVERAGE BASAL VALUES DURING 2 WEEKS OF
CONTROL PERIODS BEFORE AND AFTER

Figure 18. Sustained hypersecretion of HCl and hyperemia of the gastric mucosa of Tom during a two-week period of emotional conflict characterized by anger and resentment (center shaded bars) compared with values during the preceding and succeeding weeks (open bars).

generally to be craving support and recognition and especially vulnerable to threats to their manly assertive independence. Whether their characteristic behavior of competitive striving is related to an atavistic urge to devour an adversary can only be speculated upon, but it is striking that an accentuation of gastric acid secretion and motor activity associated with the production of gastric pain can be readily induced in ulcer patients by discussions that arouse feelings of inadequacy, frustration and resentment.

In considering the pathogenesis of peptic ulcer, many factors must be given weight including the important one of heredity, but certainly the individual's way of life and the way in which he

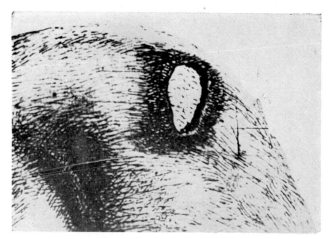

Figure 19. Ulcer experimentally produced on Tom's gastric mucosa after prolonged contact of an eroded area with his own acid gastric juice.

sees himself in relation to his situation and his fellow men are of more than passing importance (48).

Gastric Hypofunction

Gastric hypofunction is a regular accompaniment of anorexia and nausea and occurs typically following the ingestion of a noxious substance such as ipecac or copper sulfate. It also occurs when the evacuated gastric content is "unacceptable" to the duodenum in quantity, consistency, hydrogen ion concentration or osmolarity. Gastric hypofunction is clearly a protective reaction, tending as it does to limit digestion and absorption, and accompanied, as it often is, by vomiting, i.e., regurgitation of the offending substance (49, 50).

Like hyperfunction, gastric hypofunction occurs in many circumstances unconnected with alimentation. Hypofunction has been encountered typically in overwhelming situations fraught with feelings of terror, dejection and despair (Fig. 20). Long standing gastric hypofunction has been observed in depressed people and as a consequence of the accompanying anorexia, may be associated with weight loss, weakness and more or less debility.

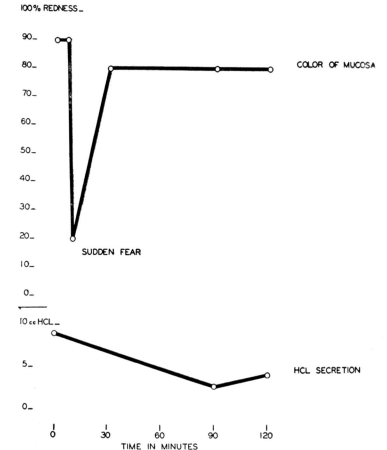

Figure 20. Transitory gastric hypofunction in Tom associated with a frightening situation.

The Colon—Mechanism of Diarrhea

The colon is subject to at least three distinguishable patterns of disturbed motility, one associated with diarrhea and two with constipation. The normal activities of the right side of the colon can be distinguished from those of the left side. The cecum and ascending colon by rhythmic peristaltic waves propel their contents through the transverse and into the descending and sigmoid colon. These latter structures facilitate the passage of feces through the usually redundant left colon by assuming a tube-like posture which results from sustained contraction of the longitudinal and circular muscles. This sequence of events characterizes the gastro-colic reflex. It is not a direct reflex but a conditioned response that occurs normally after meals, and can be trained to produce defecation at a designated time of day. The gastrocolic reflex, however, may be evoked inappropriately by symbolic stimuli, situations which elicit a passive-aggressive reaction of hostility. Diarrhea occurs when the gastro-colic reflex is too frequent or too vigorous (51). Grace and Graham considered such diarrhea as a riddance pattern (30). They found the conversation of patients sprinkled with statements expressing a desire to get rid of or dispose of troubles. (See Chapter IV.) Grace and associates studied patients with ulcerative colitis, including some with exposed portions of colonic mucous membrane (51). They found hyperemia, engorgement and increased fragility of the mucosa when sustained colonic hyperfunction of the gastrocolic reflex type was precipitated by problems of life adjustment. Indeed, in one subject whose left colon had been removed and whose cecum and a part of the ascending colon were evaginated and exposed on the abdominal wall, a full blown attack of ulcerative colitis occurred following a visit home during which he discovered that his own bedroom had been taken over by a sister. As in the case of the stomach and other tissues, it was possible through the technique of the stress interview to manipulate colonic function and to induce the characteristic pattern of the gastrocolic reflex.

Constipation

A. *Hyperfunction of the Sigmoid Colon*

During intervals between the gastrocolic reflex, the material in the left side of the colon is kneaded and dried out by forceful but non-propulsive contractions of the descending and sigmoid colon. When such activity is excessive, and particularly in the absence of adequate propulsive function, the stool becomes dry, hard and difficult to evacuate. Such "spastic constipation" is often accompanied by abdominal cramps and it may even be possible to palpate as a mass the contracted wall of the sigmoid

case of such potentially serious disorders as atrial fibrillation and ventricular tachycardia (60, 170).

Electrocardiogram

Ordinarily, when there are changes in the pattern of the electrocardiogram during exercise, the assumption is made that there is a disturbance of cardiac nutrition. In the study of Stevenson *et al.* (61), nineteen patients displayed changes in S-T segments or T waves to a degree considered significant, according to the criteria of Master, when exercise was performed during a period of stress. The same exercise on a day of relative security and relaxation produced less change in the electrocardiogram, or none at all. In all but one of the nineteen, it was possible to produce electrocardiographic changes during an interview covering pertinent personal problems and without exercise or conscious anticipation of muscular effort. This information is in keeping with the general concept that man during stress may react with his cardiovascular apparatus as if he were about to engage in strenuous muscular activity without any actual awareness of anticipating exercise (60-65).

Figure 21 illustrates changes observed in the electrocardiogram of one subject, aged thirty-two, who at the time had

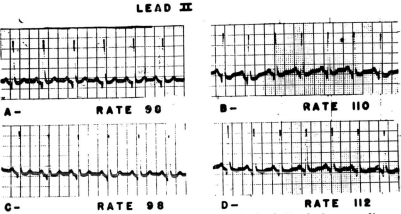

Figure 21. Marked depression of T waves in lead II of electrocardiogram immediately after exercise (B) and during discussion of anxiety about his heart (D). A and C are control tracings prior to exercise and prior to interview.

symptoms of palpitation and reduced exercise tolerance without evidence of structural heart disease except in the electrocardiogram; this was normal at rest but the T waves became inverted during exercise or during a stressful interview. Seven years later, the patient still showed no further evidence of heart disease.

The mechanisms responsible for these changes cannot be stated on the basis of the data at hand. They may include coronary ischemia or perhaps reflect stimulation of sympathetic or vagal fibers.

There is some evidence that hyperventilation may contribute to T wave inversion and that the phenomenon may be blocked by oral ingestion of potassium salts (66). Hinkle and co-workers recorded the electrocardiogram on portable tapes worn by the subject throughout the hours of a working day and found T wave inversion and S-T depression in presumably healthy subjects not only during heavy meals or unusual exertion, but also during stressful discussions (67).

Work of the Heart

Muscular effort is a familiar stimulus to cardiovascular function. On the basis of the predictability in degree and duration of changes evoked by measured amounts of exercise, various workers have devised tests of adequacy of cardiac function and of cardiac reserve.

Briefly, expected changes include increased heart rate and stroke volume accompanied by reduced peripheral vascular resistance. Exercise tolerance, which depends on the efficient balance among these three factors together with the effectiveness of pulmonary ventilation is enhanced by physical training and impaired by prolonged inactivity. The cardiovascular response to exercise is also affected to a significant extent by the individual's state of psychological adjustment. Indeed, life situations that are either consciously or unconsciously threatening to the security of the individual may induce tachycardia and an increase in stroke volume without any exercise having been undertaken (64). The experiments of Hellerstein (68-71) are particularly illuminating. The work of the heart and linked vasomotor responses of surgeons standing at an operating table were found to equal those of men engaged in heavy labor such as moving and lifting heavy objects in a steel plant. Sarnoff (72) and Katz *et al.* (73) demonstrated a close correlation between myocardial oxygen consumption and the product of the peak systolic blood pressure and heart rate. Assuming this to be valid, one can relate total body energy to the energy expenditure of the heart. While performing a surgical operation, the caloric expenditure was low, averaging 1.8 calories per minute. Yet, certain surgeons expending 1.8 calories per minute showed an estimated myocardial oxygen consumption equal to that of men doing heavy work in a steel mill. Also, foremen, as a group, started and ended the day with higher pulse rates than those engaged in greater bodily activity, but who also had less responsibility (74). These experiments indicate the unsuspected demands upon the cardiovascular apparatus of ostensibly inactive persons during periods of responsibility. Situations of pleasurable anticipation may also be associated with tachycardia and an increase in stroke volume. It is as though bodily changes were occurring in preparation for exertion, e.g., fighting, running away, or active participation in some pleasurable situation. When exercise is actually undertaken under such circumstances, the cardiovascular adaptation may be excessive or unduly prolonged during recovery, as though a much greater muscular effort had been anticipated.

The work of Wolf and Wolff (35), and later of Hickam *et al.* (75), established that variations in stroke volume and cardiac output correspond with changes in life situation and emotional state. Duncan *et al* (63, 76), related them to some of the symptoms of neurocirculatory asthenia. The possible importance of such alterations in cardiac function to patients with already damaged hearts has not been assessed. It is noteworthy, however, that the work of the heart may be increased and its efficiency affected by circumstances constituting figurative burdens. It is also evident that the work of the heart cannot be estimated with any degree of accuracy with reference only to the amount of exertion actually undertaken. If the subject is "in training," cardiovascular efficiency will be such that a relatively great load may be carried on with a minimum of work. On the other hand, in training or not, the heart may be called upon to work hard with the subject sitting or lying while discussing or contemplating some troublesome personal problem. Indeed the changes may occur without any conscious awareness of the pertinent problem.

HEMODYNAMIC ADJUSTMENTS
Increased Peripheral Flow

The hemodynamic changes appropriate to situations requiring an increased peripheral circulation, such as anemia, vitamin deficiencies, arteriovenous shunts and hyperthyroidism, include tachycardia, increased stroke volume, and a lowering of peripheral resistance. It is well known that the same adjustments occur temporarily during vigorous muscular effort. They may also occur in anticipation of such an effort as before running a race. Indeed there may be an increase in peripheral blood flow in emotionally charged situations where there is no conscious contemplation of muscular activity. It is as if the regulatory mechanism in man, appropriate to an earlier period of evolutionary development, were involved, somewhat inappropriately, in the present day environment. Such "as if" reactions have been discussed elsewhere (77).

Systemic Hypertension

It has been shown with appropriate documentation, that hemodynamic changes productive of elevated arterial pressure, reduced renal blood flow (Fig. 22) and increased blood viscosity occur as a part of an individual's adaptation to problems and challenges in his daily life (78-80). Special attention has been directed to two contrasting patterns of hemodynamic adjustment that occur alike in hypertensive and normotensive individuals under stress. One pattern appears to be identical with the "exercise" pattern, which is characterized by an increase in blood pressure attributable to a rise in stroke volume without elevation of peripheral vascular resistance. The other pattern resembles that encountered in injury or hemorrhage. It is characterized by an increase in blood pressure attributable to an elevation in peripheral resistance without a rise in stroke volume. When observed during interviews that deal with pertinent personal conflicts, the "exercise" pattern was manifest when emotional disturbance was relatively overt, Figure 23, while the "high resistance" pattern was more often encountered with a

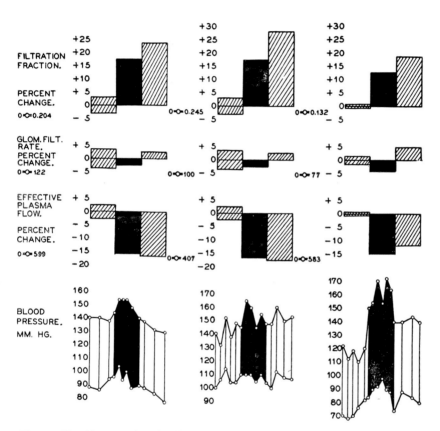

Figure 22. Changes in the blood pressure and renal hemodynamics in representative subjects. The first section of cross-hatching represents the range of variation of three separate control periods. The mean value in each instance is shown at the left of the scale as $0 \rightleftharpoons$. The solid black column represents the average change during the periods of stressful interview, and the last cross-hatched column shows the average change in the postinterview periods. Note the evidence of renal vasoconstriction during the stressful period.

calm exterior and evidence of suppression or repression of emotion (Fig. 24). It was of particular interest that both patterns elicited under circumstances of emotional conflict, were associated

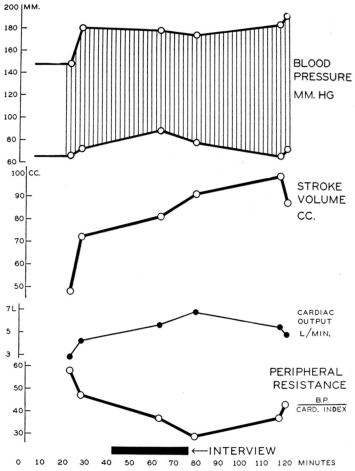

Figure 23. Cardiovascular reactions during frankly expressed anxiety. Note the decrease in peripheral resistance during rise in blood pressure, with increased stroke volume and cardiac output.

with a decrease in renal blood flow and an elevation of filtration fraction and renal vascular resistance.

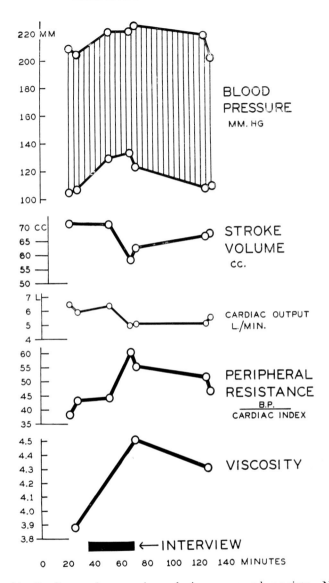

Figure 24. Cardiovascular reactions during repressed anxiety. Note the sharply increased peripheral resistance and viscosity during the rise in blood pressure, with a diminishing stroke volume and cardiac output.

In essential hypertension, there occurs a sustained increase in peripheral resistance without a rise in stroke volume. During blood loss, as in donors for transfusion, an increase has been observed in peripheral resistance without increased cardiac output but with the maintenance, or even elevation, of blood pressure. Such changes have also been seen to occur in subjects volunteering as transfusion donors but before any blood was withdrawn (60). These changes, of course, are typical of those encountered in essential hypertension and they may also be seen as overcorrective responses following the injection of hypotensive drugs, or upon assuming the recumbent position after an episode of postural hypotension. Psychiatrists have for years pointed out that patients with essential hypertension are psychologically poised for combat but that the aggressive action is unconsciously and powerfully restrained (81). The mechanisms of the vascular apparatus responsible for raising the blood pressure in humans in response to symbolic stimuli were not impaired by thoracolumbar or even "total" sympathectomy. Either the "exercise" or "high resistance" pattern might still occur, although no longer was there evidence of associated reduction in renal blood flow. It is conceivable that the loss of renal vasoconstrictor activity may protect the kidneys and thereby have a salutary effect on the course of essential hypertension. Perhaps, it may be a factor in the apparent increased survival of sympathectomized patients even without notable reduction of arterial pressure (82).

There is insufficient evidence to conclude that essential hypertension occurs in a suitably susceptible subject as part of a cardiovascular adjustment, as if in preparation for combat with threatened blood loss. Nevertheless, the fact remains that the appropriate hemodynamic mechanisms are connected with, and capable of reacting to, neural connections in the interpretive areas of the brain.

The significance of all these findings is not clear but in any case, it appears that stressful life experiences are sufficiently prominent among stimuli elevating arterial pressure to warrant their serious consideration in the clinical management of patients with essential hypertension. The evidence of emotional restraint and the calm exterior often displayed by these patients make it necessary for the physician to exercise special diligence and skill in uncovering meaningful life experiences and the attitudes and reactions associated with them.

A study of personality adjustment among the patients with hypertension did not delineate any characteristic personality "type", but yielded strikingly similar data as regards values, attitudes, and way of life. By and large the hypertensive subjects had grown up feeling that they must excel but at the same time avoid conflict or too vigorous self-assertion. These strivings, often opposed as they were, led frequently to dilemmas and were manifest by wary, tentative, and non-committal attitudes with respect to important interpersonal relations and major endeavors in life.

In a published series, 12 per cent of hypertensive patients under psychotherapy lost all evidences of hypertension. Although one cannot infer that the therapy was responsible for the change in blood pressure these individuals did appear to have developed a more confident and relaxed approach to life, a more optimistic outlook, and an improved capacity for self-assertion (60).

Availability of Lipids as Fuel for Strenuous Effort

It is easier to produce sustained hyperlipemia in man by starvation than by feeding. This finding may be explained by the pressing need to conserve glucose during starvation because nervous tissue cannot metabolize other products. The muscles, however, and other bodily tissues, can use fat for fuel as readily as glucose. The mechanism responsible for lipid mobilization involves sympathetic nerve impulses and the evidence of Seifter *et al* (83), would implicate the pituitary. Fat must also be metabolized in preference to glucose during strenuous muscular effort. There is not sufficient glucose in the body, or in glycogen stores, to support the muscular effort involved in stoking a furnace or skiing cross-country Therefore, as in starvation, the muscles must rely on fat as a source of energy. Here again, as shown in the work of Naughton and Balke, there occurs an elevation in serum cholesterol and lipids (84).

Coronary Heart Disease

The mechanisms responsible for coronary artherosclerosis are still obscure. So is the relationship of atherosclerosis to myocardial infarction and of myocardial infarction to the mechanisms of death. The pathogenesis of coronary atherosclerosis appears to be related in some way to lipid metabolism and especially the serum concentration of cholesterol.

Numerous investigators have shown that stressful life experiences are capable of evoking hypercholesterolemia (85). Several workers have studied the serum concentration of cholesterol and lipids in students before, during and after the stress of examinations. All of them, including Thomas and Murphy (86), Wertlake *et al.* (87), Grundy and Griffin (88), and Dreyfuss and Czaczkes (89), found higher values during the stressful periods than otherwise. Dreyfuss also measured the clotting time and found it accelerated in thirty-six medical students on the morning of a final examination in medicine. In other studies reported by Groen (90), Groover (91), Friedman and Rosenman (92), and Hammarsten and associates (93), there was evidence that the lipid regulating mechanisms are responsive to situational stress. The latter studies were undertaken on twelve men ranging in age from thirty to seventy. Each gave well documented evidence of a previous myocardial infarction. These individuals were followed at weekly intervals with chemical determination of serum cholesterol, lipid phosphorus and lipoproteins, as estimated by the ultracentrifugal technique. At the same time, each subject kept a written record of everything consumed each day at meals, and between meals. The dietary records were later analyzed and roughly quantitated in terms of caloric content and proportion of fat, carbohydrate and protein in the diet. In addition, the subjects were weighed each week and carefully interviewed concerning events of the week and their attitudes and reactions to potentially stressful situations. Following the interview, the investigator recorded a judgment concerning the presence or absence of significant stress during the week and an estimate of its degree. These data were, of course, gathered and recorded entirely separately from the chemical measurements. Later correlation showed that unusually high cholesterol concentration, more than 15 per cent above the mean for any individual in the study, correlated with a high degree of significance, with periods that had been separately judged as especially stressful. Similar correlation was found in the lipoproteins of the SF 0-12 and the SF 12-20 fractions. More recently, these data have been reinforced by studies of four subjects on balance regimens in a metabolic ward. During the period of rigidly maintained uniform diet and exercise, variations in the concentration of the serum cholesterol of 15 to 40 per cent were observed, amounting to nearly 100 mg per cent (Fig. 25). A high degree of statistical significance was noted when periods

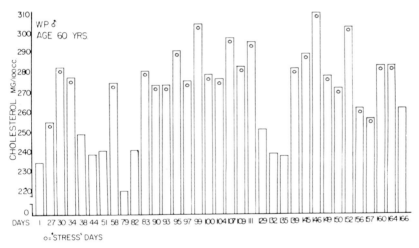

Figure 25. Changes in serum concentration of cholesterol in a subject on a metabolic ward during several months of constant diet and exercise. Twenty-five days independently judged as stressful are marked with circle. (Mean cholesterol concentration: 283, with S.D.=12.5. Mean concentration on ten non-stressful days: 242, with S.D.=10.3.)

of cholesterol elevation were correlated with periods of separately judged emotional stress (94). Further documentation was available from short-term experiments in which the patients were subjected to stressful interviews concerning their significant personal conflicts. In control interviews covering neutral topics no elevations of serum cholesterol were observed. Following an hour of stressful discussion, however, an increase in the serum cholesterol occurred in five out of six times (Fig. 26). Other workers

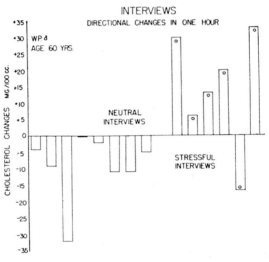

Figure 26. Comparison of short-term changes in serum cholesterol during neutral and stressful interviews in the subject illustrated in Figure 25.

have studied changes in the serum concentration of free fatty acids in relation to stressful experiences (95, 96).

The studies of Hammarsten, and his associates, indicated that patients with coronary artery disease were oriented to life along the line of effort, of doing things "the hard way" (93). These patients place an especially high value on doing things "on their own" and being solely responsible for their activities and experiences. Like Sisyphus, they appeared to be continually carrying a burden and never quite getting it to the top of the hill or the resting place. Moreover, the occurrence of coronary attacks appeared to correlate with periods when the individuals were carrying an especially heavy emotional load with relatively little support from those about them. It may be that the mechanisms that govern the concentration of serum lipid are brought into play in the face of demand for effort that is figurative as well as literal. The possibility that any such changes are actually related to the mechanisms of coronary atherosclerosis is entirely speculative. Moreover, it should be borne in mind that not only are the mechanisms regulating the concentration of serum lipids and cholesterol unknown at present, but the significance of the relation of serum concentration of these substances to the integrity of arteries is equally obscure. Indeed, the extent to which the presence of atherosclerosis determines vascular accidents is also unknown.

The opinion of many present-day investigators is reflected in the following editorial comment of Oliver and Boyd in the *British Heart Journal*: "The remarkable social and economic changes of the century are undoubtedly stressful to some people. Increasing stress might favor the development of clinical coronary disease by disturbing normal endocrine balance and thus influencing both cholesterol metabolism and the coagulation and fibrinolytic systems. Similarly, long continued environmental stress might disturb the autonomic control of the coronary arteries" (97). Convincing evidence to support such notions is still lacking, but several clinical studies of groups of patients with coronary artery disease would tend to support them. Thus, Friedman and Rosenman found higher serum cholesterol concentrations, a far greater incidence of arcus senilis and a vastly increased incidence of evidence of coronary artery disease in subjects classified as oriented toward competitive activities with deadlines, as compared with anxious but noncompetitive people or with more passive subjects (92). Russek reported similar findings among coronary patients (98), and Dreyfuss (99), and Weiss *et al.* (100), observed special situational stresses as antecedent events to episodes of coronary occlusion. Schneider and associates (101) followed carefully fifty patients with known coronary artery disease and fifty matched controls. They found less sinus arrythmia in the coronary patients than in controls of comparable age, but nevertheless a greater lability of heart rate, including bradycardia in response to minor alerting stimuli. The same group of coronary patients was found by Hampton and associates (102) to display a greater variability of fibrinogen concentration in blood serum than the presumably healthy controls. Bruhn and Adsett (103) found this same group to be less capable of achieving satisfaction and social approval through effort than the control group. The relationship of social and cultural mobility to the occurrence of coronary heart disease has been illuminated by the studies of Wardwell *et al.* (165), Christenson and Hinkle (74) and Syme *et al.* (166). The evidence relating psychological phenomena to disease of the heart and blood vessels though fragmentary, is sufficiently promising to warrant a great deal more serious interest on the part of physiologists and clinicians.

GENITO-URINARY SYSTEM
A. The Kidneys

While the lungs are concerned with two way exchanges with the environment, the kidneys are responsible only for maintaining internal equilibrium by eliminating certain substances, including especially water, inorganic salts, acids and nitrogenous wastes. The control of renal function is exerted through the behavior of arteries and arterioles and through the chemical constituents of the blood which act on sensitive receptors in the kidney tubules. Most of these mechanisms, renal blood flow, glomerular filtration rate, renal vascular resistance and tubular function with respect to the absorption of sodium, chloride, calcium, and nitrogen have been shown to be responsive to the highest integrative functions of the brain (104).

With respect to the circulatory phenomena in the kidney Pfeiffer *et al* (105, 79), have shown that in hypertensive subjects and certain other susceptible humans, renal blood flow may be significantly reduced and vascular resistance increased during "stress interviews," with accompanying elevation of arterial pressure. It is especially interesting that the circulatory changes in the kidney outlasted the period of induced hypertension. The excretion of water and electrolytes was the subject of study by Schottstaedt *et al.* (106-109), who demonstrated striking diuresis in association with attitudes characterized by anxiety and aggressive feelings. Retention of salt and water accompanied mental concentration or attitudes of immobility or withdrawal. The most striking retention was found among those suffering from depression. The magnitude of water and salt retention in some cardiac patients during episodes of depression was such as to precipitate the manifestations of congestive heart failure. Luetscher (110) documented in women under emotionally stressful circumstances an increase in urinary excretion of aldosterone associated with sodium retention and the appearance of peripheral edema. An interesting characteristic of renal excretion found typical of hypertensive subjects is the relatively great and prompt diuretic and natriuretic response to an intravenously administered salt load. Welmer and Groen demonstrated that the prompt, exaggerated natriuresis reflected the psychologic 'set' of the individual and was unrelated t othe mechanism of the hypertension itself (167).

B. The Bladder

Hyperfunction of the bladder musculature manifested as urinary frequency, and hypofunction manifested as urinary retention were found to be associated with opposite attitudes vis-a-vis troublesome life situations (111, 112). Ripley and Wolf (113) studied patients with elusive (Hunner's) ulcer of the bladder associated with painful frequency and sometimes bleeding, and found that exacerbations correlated with periods of frustration and intense hostility and resentment, usually unexpressed, and often masked by a facade of sweetness and tractability. The painful state was elucidated by McLellan and Goodell (114) who showed that sensitivity to pain in the bladder mucosa was greatly increased when the membrane was hyperemic and engorged, a characteristic of bladder hyperfunction with urinary frequency.

Stubborn urinary retention was identified in response to difficult life situations when the dominant attitude of the patient included intense fear, often completely repressed, and discouragement or dejection. Reversible urinary retention amounting to 1800 ml of water was encountered among American soldiers under the terrifying circumstances of combat in the Pacific in World War II (115). Often, bladder function was re-

stored after removal of the soldier from the danger zone and
with the aid of reassuring psychotherapy at times supplemented
by intravenous injections of the hypnotic sodium amytal. In
most instances the accompanying psychological picture was one
of hysteria and denial of conflict, the emotional turmoil being

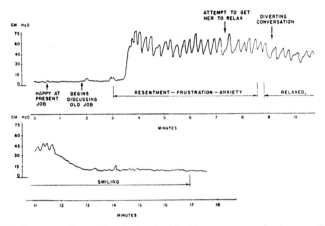

Figure 27. Sharp and sustained rise in bladder pressure during conflict with
anxiety, followed by a return to the initial base line during relaxation and
relative security.

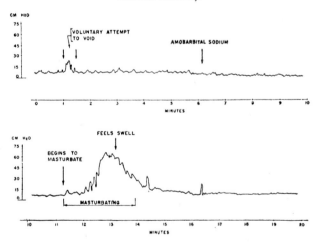

Figure 28. Urinary retention with low intracystic pressure in a subject whose
bladder had not been emptied for more than twelve hours. A vigorous
contractile wave occurred during masturbation following intravenous injection of amobarbital sodium.

brought to light only after sodium amytal had been administered.

In civilian life, urinary retention with hypotonia of the bladder attributable to stress-evoking situations was encountered more frequently among females than males. Measurements made with a cystometric device revealed a striking reduction in responsiveness of the bladder musculature to stretch, and hence a reduced awareness of the full bladder and a blunted urge to void (116, 117). During experimental sessions in the laboratory, it was found possible to manipulate bladder motility by focussing the patient's attention on either troublesome or reassuring topics (Figs. 27 & 28).

C. The Female Reproductive Tract

Numerous gynecological disorders have been attributed in part to stress-evoking situations. Among these perhaps the toxemia of pregnancy has received the greatest attention of investigators (118). The mechanisms responsible for the manifestations of toxemia of pregnancy involve the kidney more prominently than the reproductive organs.

Sterility has been linked to emotional conflicts and tensions by certain physicians since antiquity, but it has been difficult to gather more than anecdotal evidence on this important phenomenon. Uterine dysrhythmia resulting in difficult labor, or, in the absence of pregnancy, dysmenorrhea, have been observed in association with important emotional conflicts, and have been subjected to experimental study (Mann) (119-121).

Other abdominal discomforts related to pelvic structures have been studied by Duncan and Taylor (122) who found evidence of painful vascular engorgement associated with emotional conflicts, especially those involving sexual behavior. In other investigations (123, 124), the mucosa of the vagina was found like so many other tissues, to become either hyperemic and moist on the one hand, or pale and dry on the other, in association with changing emotions, moods and preoccupations. Sustained hyperemia occurring under circumstances of sexual deprivation was found to be accompanied by excessive secretion of the vaginal glands, and complaints of leucorrhoea. Pallor and dryness on the other hand accompanied depressive reactions and attitudes of withdrawal.

THE ENDOCRINE GLANDS AND METABOLISM
A. Diabetes

Although the complex chain of metabolic events that characterizes diabetes has not been fully elucidated, it is clear that some of the changes, salt and water diuresis and elevations in blood glucose concentration and the occurrence of ketonemia and ketonuria may be greatly accentuated in diabetic patients when they are exposed to stress-evoking circumstances without alteration in diet or muscular activity (125). By such means, episodes of ketosis and near-coma have been induced inadvertently and then experimentally in hospitalized diabetics whose dietary intake and muscular activity were held constant.

A failure to utilize glucose by skeletal muscles and other bodily structures which are not glucose dependent, and increased production of ketone bodies by the liver is a well recognized adaptation to starvation. Thus being accompanied as it is with

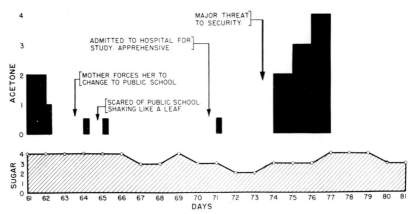

Figure 29. Association of glycosuria and urinary acetone secretion with significant events in the life situation of a 15-year-old girl. An episode of ketoacidosis lasting three days was induced while the patient was in the hospital on constant diet, exercise and insulin. The acidosis cleared following strong reassurance and emotional support without change in diet or insulin.

diuresis as the body increases its fat catabolism, starvation resembles the diabetic state. It may therefore, be significant that Hinkle *et al.*, studying diabetic patients from the standpoint of their attitudes and patterns of life adjustment found, especially among juvenile diabetics but also among many who acquired the disease in middle age, a prominent though often suppressed or repressed conviction of having been "starved" of maternal love (126 thru 129). The tendency to substitute calories for emotional nourishment has been well recognized by physicians for centuries and it may be that through emotional deprivation a figurative starvation contributes in some measure to the complex pathological process of diabetes. In diabetic patients admitted to the hospital with glycosuria but no ketosis and maintained in balance on a constant regimen of insulin, diet and exercise, ketoacidosis was induced in association with stressful events and dispelled after reassurance, without any change in the regimen (130) (Fig. 29).

B. The Pituitary Gland

It has been suspected that the accentuation of the diabetic state by stress-evoking situations is mediated through the pituitary gland and its growth hormone. The pituitary in turn is known to be susceptible to influence from the nervous system via the hypothalamus. Conceivably, other trophic hormones of the pituitary including thyroid stimulating hormone, adrenocorticotrophic hormone and follicle stimulating hormone may influence their respective target glands in response to impulses from those parts of the brain which are concerned with the interpretation of life experiences. These important avenues, still incompletely explored, offer a challenging welcome to the investigator.

The pituitary-adrenal axis may be involved in the "depletion syndromes" which occur, for example, following prolonged attacks of vascular headache of the migraine type. In this connection, it is interesting that administration of ACTH by intravenous drip has been found helpful in shortening the period of "depletion" and restoring energy (131).

C. The Thyroid Gland

The activity of the thyroid gland as reflected by the concentration of protein-bound iodine in the blood was long thought to vary little from a level characteristic for each individual. Hetzel, however, was able to adduce evidence of both hyper- and hypofunction of the thyroid as reflected by protein-bound iodine in human subjects exposed to stress-evoking life situations (132). Increases of as much as 100 per cent were recorded in some patients in as short a space as an hour after the start of a stress interview. Especially impressive elevations of protein-bound iodine were found to accompany vascular headache of the migraine type. Hetzel and coworkers have extended their findings in humans (133) and have demonstrated changes in thyroid hormone secretion in association with stress producing circumstances in animals with exteriorized glands (134).

Clinical hyperthyroidism has often been considered to have been precipitated by life crises (135) and some workers (136) have identified a type of individual susceptible to hyperthyroidism, women, especially, with a strong psychological need to care for others.

Pertinent is the fact that the incidence of hyperthyroidism in Norway (137) during the first year of World War II (1941) was twice that of the previous year, or five-fold the incidence of the year 1934. Most of the patients were women. A striking rise also occurred in Denmark and Holland, whereas neutral Sweden exhibited no change.

Hypothyroidism has been less frequently attributed to situational difficulties but the mental and emotional changes characteristic of reduced thyroid function are familiar to physicians.

D. The Adrenal Gland

The monumental studies of Selye (138) have implicated the adrenal cortex in a host of physiological disturbances and tissue reactions in animals. Acute changes in plasma concentration and urinary excretion of corticoid have been observed in man under a variety of symbolic stimuli (139) and there may be modifications of the diurinal patterns of plasma corticosteroid concentrations (140). The most familiar changes in endocrine function that occur in response to troublesome life situations involve the adrenal medulla and other sources of catecholamines (141). Levi and von Euler have made extensive studies of epinephrin and nor-epinephrin excretion in human subjects in a variety of emotionally significant situations, and have concluded that the acute changes in catechols correlate more closely with the intensity than with the type of pleasant or unpleasant emotional experience (168).

Nutrition

A. *Anorexia Nervosa*

Severe malnutrition may occur when there is adequate nourishment available if for some reason a patient cannot bring himself to eat. Anorexia leading to malnutrition is a familiar feature of severe depression, but such malnutrition may occur in apparently serene and highly energetic subjects, usually young women as part of the syndrome of anorexia nervosa (142). There is rarely a true anorexia in this condition but rather a fear of eating or an unexplainable compulsion not to eat. The emotional conflicts associated with this illness are characteristically deep-seated and complex, not infrequently of a sexual nature involving ambivalent feelings towards the subject's father. Food may play a prominent part in the patient's preoccupations and there may be dreams of eating or preparing food, and yet an inability to eat upon awakening. Associated with the wasting and and weight loss which are characteristic of the condition, there is usually amenorrhea resulting from impaired secretion of pituitary gonadotropin and at times evidence of hypofunction of other glands (143).

B. *Obesity*

Recent studies indicate that obesity may result from disturbed fat metabolism as well as from overeating. It has become customary, therefore, to refer to two types of obesity- nutritional and metabolic (144). Such two types can be readily separated when obesity is experimentally induced in animals (145). In humans, however, the indication is that obesity results in most cases from a combination of nutritional and metabolic factors. Psychiatrists have long been interested in the psychological basis for overeating. The studies of Stunkard have been particularly illuminating. He found among many obese patients a compulsive need to eat at night, especially when lonely (146).

This distinctive eating pattern of obese patients, the "night-eating syndrome," is characterized by nocturnal hyperphagia, insomnia and morning anorexia. The syndrome was present in twenty of twenty-five obese patients treated in a special study clinic and in none of thirty-eight non-obese subjects. Patients manifesting the syndrome had great difficulty in losing weight and experienced a high incidence of complications in their attempts. Stunkard found that the extent of night eating reflects closely the emotional state of the patient and may serve as an index of the success of psychotherapeutic measures.

Stunkard also found that his obese patients were far less active than non-obese subjects, and expended relatively few calories in physical activity. In another study he found a diminished appreciation of gastric sensations suggesting that a local disturbance may contribute to a general denial of satiety (144). The area in the ventro medial nucleus of the hypothalamus which is concerned with satiety is responsive to the concentration of glucose in the blood. Its firing may be affected indirectly by situational factors which alter the concentration of glucose. Also, neural impulses acting directly on this area, as inhibitory or excitatory influences from the highest integrative levels of the brain, may modulate eating behavior (145).

In considering the therapy of obesity, Stunkard calls attention to an important complication, the dieting depression, a severe reaction to voluntary food restriction. The depression may be serious and may follow an initial period of elation consequent upon successful restriction of food intake and weight loss (147). Whatever subsequent studies may reveal about the etiology of obesity, it is clear that therapy limited to dieting and without consideration of the patient as a person and his problems of life adjustment, is insufficient (148).

THE CENTRAL NERVOUS SYSTEM

While the central nervous system appears to be importantly implicated in all of the disturbances herein reviewed, there are certain disorders, for example seizures, which are classified by convention as "neurological." Since ancient times the dramatic and often alarming manifestations of a grand mal seizure have been associated in the minds of men, with uncontrollable rage. In a careful study of patients with recurrent seizures, Barker was able to correlate exacerbations of the illness with periods of situational conflict engendering suppressed rage (149, 150). It was even possible experimentally to evoke seizures in suitably susceptible subjects by a stress interview while an electroencephalographic recording was being made (151). (See Fig. 46, Ch. IV.) Not only grand mal but also petit mal was so studied, and even attacks of narocolepsy were induced by discussion of troublesome topics and with corroborative electroencephalographic documentation.

Other neurological diseases, multiple sclerosis, myasthenia gravis and paralysis agitans have been thought by many to be subject to modification by meaningful life experiences. Detailed studies are lacking, but physicians commonly associate exacerbations and remissions of these disorders with changing attitudes and reactions in patients. Indeed the full blown manifestations of Parkinson's Syndrome have been observed to appear, de novo, following a particularly terrifying experience, such as an artillery barrage (152).

THE SKIN

Of all of the organs of the body, with the possible exception of the respiratory apparatus, the skin has the greatest exposure to the environment. It is concerned with the regulation of body temperature and its rich vascular supply is responsive to a variety of forces in its external and internal environment (153, 154). One very dramatic example of the participation of the skin in the body's adaptations was provided by an experiment by Graham (155, 156).

The reactivity of the minute vessels in the skin of a subject's two arms was tested according to the method of di Palma, Reynolds and Foster (157). After preliminary measurements, the left arm was struck. Immediately, the resistance of the vessels to dilatation was decreased. The same change in vascular tone was noted in the other arm which was not struck. The injured left arm gradually returned to its former state; the right arm recovered a little sooner. Shortly, the experiment was repeated, except that now a sham blow was delivered, i.e., instead of bringing the ferule down onto the forearm it was stopped just short of the surface. The capillaries of the left arm behaved just as they had before, though no injury was inflicted. This time the right arm did not respond. Gradually the left arm returned to its former state. Soon the whole procedure was repeated except that the subject was told that a sham blow was about to descend. After this anticipated sham blow, no change in capillary tone occurred (Fig. 30).

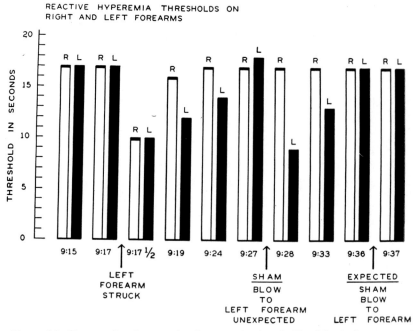

Figure 30. Changes in the reactive hyperemia threshold of both forearms of a healthy man in response to real and feigned blows to the left forearm.

A second experiment concerned a subject with "hives." A control measurement of the resistance of the capillaries of his skin to dilatation was made. Then, instead of striking his forearm with a ferule, Graham introduced as a topic for discussion a painful family situation, causing the patient to feel as though he were being struck. "Just thinking about the things they did to me" was his answer when asked about his attitude at this moment. Simultaneously the capillaries of the forearm behaved as though he actually had been struck; their resistance to dilatation decreased and wheals, or hives, developed. Thus the bodily pattern set in motion by a blow from a ferule in the first instance

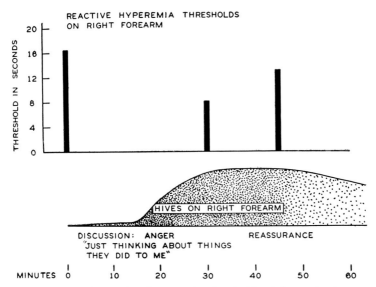

Figure 31. Lowered reactive hyperemia threshold while urticaria was developing, with return toward normal as lesions ceased to appear.

was displayed also against a symbolic blow (Fig. 31). While the subject revealed his attitude as that of "taking a beating," which he could not avoid, his skin actually reacted as though it were being struck.

In a third experiment at a later date, another subject's skin was tested as regards its reactions to mechanical stroking, and to very small amounts of histamine and pilocarpine. Her skin in preliminary tests did not react to these noxious procedures in the amounts given. She was then exposed to the discussion of a disturbing topic which caused her to feel abused and angry and yet helpless to do anything about it. At the height of her troubled state, a repetition of the stimuli that a few minutes before had produced no effect, now caused a vigorous urticarial reaction. This subject had become vulnerable, during discussion of the painful topic, to unrelated assaults and previously non-noxious stimuli. Soon thereafter, following words of reassurance, she returned to her first state and in an additional test her skin again did not react to the stroking, histamine or pilocarpine (Fig. 32).

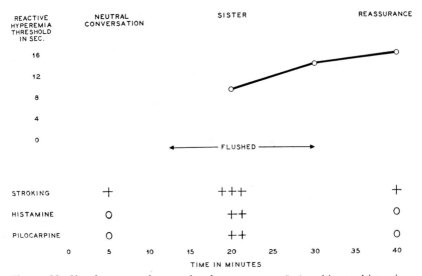

Figure 32. Simultaneous changes in the response of the skin to histamine, to pilocarpine, and to stroking during a stressful interview with a woman patient. (Histamine acid phosphate 0.001 per cent, and pilocarpine hydrochloride 1 per cent at only 10 microamperes for two minutes over 1 square centimeter.) There was no response to physiological saline applied in the same way before, during and after the period of stress.

Eczema

Relation Between Life Situations and Symptoms

In twenty-six of thirty-one patients studied by Graham, there was established a clear-cut temporal correlation between life

events which the patient recognized as emotionally disturbing
and exacerbations of eczema (158). The correlation applied not
only to major attacks, but also to relatively minor episodes of
itching and scratching lasting for only an hour or two.

The life situations which were correlated with attacks of
eczema varied, but the patients' attitudes at such times were essentially similar. They considered themselves to be frustrated.

Mild attacks of eczema occurred in circumstances usually

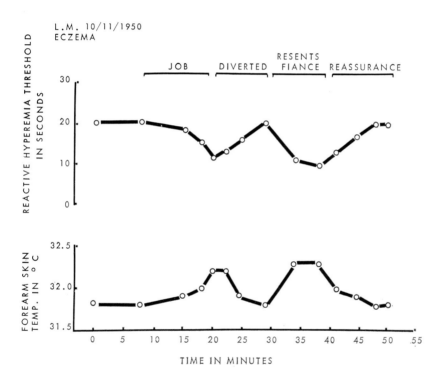

Figure 33. Cutaneous vasodilatation, involving both the minute vessels and
the arterioles, on the forearm skin during stressful interview. Exacerbations
of her exzema were found to occur in response to certain features of her
job and to some aspects of her fiances' behavior. It will be seen that mention
of each of these subjects provoked vascular changes.

called "embarrassing." The word embarrass implies some influence that impedes thought, speech or action, and may be used
with reference not only to persons but to the things they plan

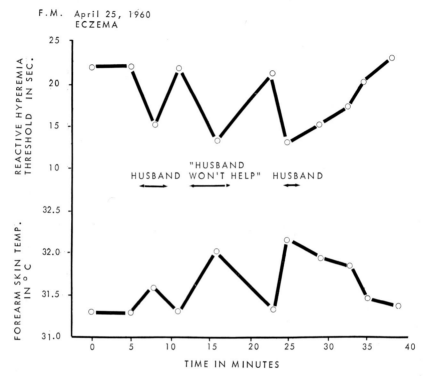

Figure 34. Cutaneous vascular changes on the volar surface of the forearm during a stressful interview. Each time her husband was mentioned, there was a fall in the reactive hyperemia threshold and a rise in skin temperature, indicating decreased minute vessel tone combined with arteriolar dilatation.

or desire to do" (*Webster's New Collegiate Dictionary,* 1956), and one prominent feature of such situations is the inability to think of a way to retaliate.

In fifteen experiments on fourteen subjects, there was increase in skin temperature of at least 0.3 degree (indicating dilatation of arterioles) when the subjects were discussing those events in their lives known to have been associated with exacerbations of the dermatitis. Minute vessel tone was decreased as indicated by a fall in the reactive hyperemia threshold of at least five seconds. Pain threshold was also lowered in the area of itchy skin.

Even if "spontaneous" itching did not occur, light scratching of the skin by a pin was reported to be felt as itchier than the same scratching during control periods of greater tranquillity, in which there was no cutaneous vasodilatation. Typical experiments are illustrated in Figures 33, 34, and 35.

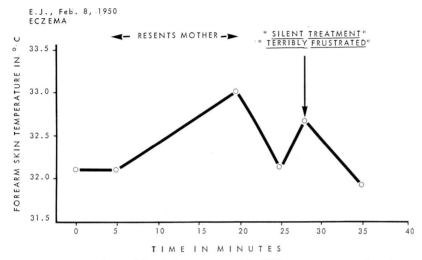

Figure 35. Interview with adult woman with lifelong eczema and asthma. The reactive hyperemia threshold could not be measured because of skin damage. Discussion of her mother's treatment of her when she was a child resulted in arteriolar dilatation.

Figure 36 illustrates a control experiment. With the deliberate avoidance of disturbing topics during an interview, significant cutaneous vascular changes did not occur.

Scratching by patients with eczema cannot be simply explained as an effort to relieve itching, as many authors have noted. Self-punishment was in many of the patients a very important element in scratching, so that the latter was much more intense and prolonged than seemed to be appropriate to the intensity of the itching. This aspect seemed to be of major significance in at least half of the patients, and was of some importance in all of them. Their attitudes were expressed by such statements as "I scratch until I've punished myself enough," "I take it out on myself," and "I stop when I've done myself enough damage."

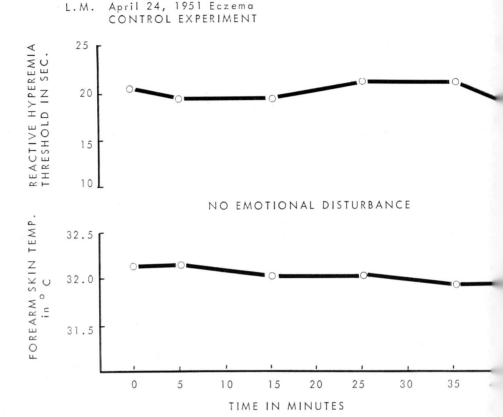

Figure 36. Lack of cutaneous vascular change in subject illustrated in Figure 33 during interview conducted in a reassuring way, with avoidance of stressful topics.

There is, in addition, a definitely pleasurable aspect of itching and scratching on which several authors have commented. Two of the patients in the present series mentioned this as important. One woman said, "When I'm scratching, when the itching has ceased, it's the biggest thrill I could encounter," and also remarked that she was "more interested" in her itching than in sexual intercourse. One man referred to the "diabolical pleasure" he got from scratching.

Finally, many patients stated that they scratched sometimes when there was no itching, at times of "tension." In such circumstances, it seemed to be comparable to table-tapping or any other habitual tension-relieving activity in individuals without skin disease.

Vasodilatation and increased itchiness appeared to be closely related, but the patients in this series seemed to be driven to scratch themselves to an extent somewhat greater than could be accounted for by their itching.

Sebum Secretion and Acne Vulgaris

Acne occurs most typically in early adolescence, a period characterized by general upheaval in glandular, psychological and social adjustments. The development of pustules seems to be related in some way to the quantity of sebum secreted, and the freedom with which it gains access to the surface of the skin through the ducts of the sebaceous glands.

Thus, as a part of an inquiry into the mechanism of acne vulgaris (159, 160) roughly quantitative measurements of hu-

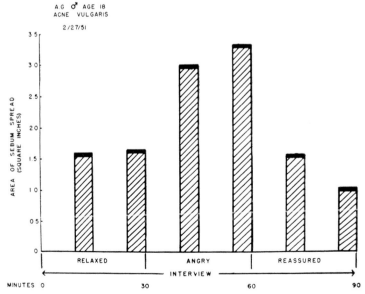

Figure 37. Increase in facial sebum output during a stressful interview inducing anger in an 18-year-old male with acne vulgaris.

man sebum were made by applying the end of a glass rod to the skin surface under standard conditions to obtain a specimen of sebum. This could then be assayed by measuring planimetrically the area of spread of the sebum as a film in a monomolecular oil layer on water.

Washing the skin with soap and water or with alcohol and ether eliminated surface sebum and yielded zero readings. After initial washing, the reaccumulation of sebum occurred gradually, reaching approximately the pre-wash level within sixty minutes. During periods of tranquillity, an approximately constant facial sebum output was maintained. Observations on patients with acne vulgaris showed that during induced reactions of anger, sebum output was increased two-to-five fold (Fig. 37).

The outstanding pattern of emotional response in a series of patients with acne vulgaris was intense anger followed by depression and remorse. A close correlation was found between these phasic emotional reactions, alterations in seborrhea, and increase in the number of acne lesions (Fig. 38).

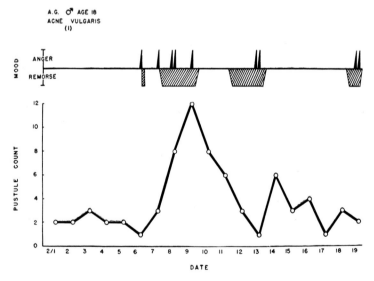

Figure 38. Comparison of the occurrence of phasic changes in mood from anger to remorse, with the daily pustule count on the face of an 18-year-old male with acne vulgaris.

Inflammatory Reactions

The participation of various levels of the nervous system in adaptive responses involving inflammation following a standard noxious thermal stimulus was analyzed (161, 162, 7, 8, 163).

Vasodilatation in the skin due to neural activity confined to a peripheral sensory nerve (the axon reflex) was accompanied by a striking lowering of pain threshold in the reddened area. Moreover, the vulnerability of the skin to noxious stimulation was enhanced during the axon reflex as manifest by the occurrence of greater tissue damage following a standard heat stimulus. Figure 39 illustrates the apparatus used.

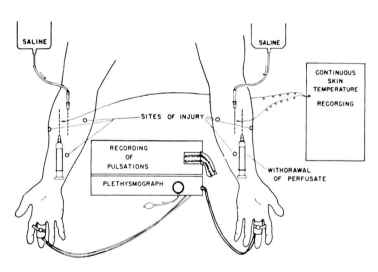

Figure 39. The arrangement of apparatus and recording devices for perfusion of two arms, collection of perfusate, recording of finger pulsations and measurement and recording of skin temperature. Four number 20, 2 in. long perforate needles* were used. This is our adaptation of the method of Fox and Hilton (46).

Antidromic impulses in sensory nerves were found to result in the elaboration of neurokinin, referred to before under headache, a powerful dilator of small blood vessels and a substance

*These needles were specially made for us by Becton, Dickinson Company, Rutherford, New Jersey

which lowers pain threshold (7, 8).

Vasodilator activity in the skin, integrated at the level of the brain stem as in thermoregulatory reflexes, was also accompanied by increased sensitivity to pain and increased tissue vulnerability to graded noxious stimuli. Cooling of the skin of the forearm reflexly by cooling the feet and legs in a tub of water was associated with elevation of pain threshold and lowered vulnerability to the noxious heat stimulus (162). The size of an axon reflex flare following local injection of histamine was greatly reduced by this maneuver.

Effects of Hypnosis

Vasomotor effects were also elicited as a result of neural activity at the highest integrative levels of the nervous system. Such effects were induced in human subjects by hypnosis as follows (163).

Thirteen subjects were hypnotized in forty experiments. As soon as a state of moderate to deep hypnosis had been established it was suggested that one arm was either "normal," or that it was "anaesthetic," "numb," "wooden," and devoid of sensation. It was then suggested that the other arm was painful, burning, damaged, and exceedingly sensitive, i.e., "vulnerable." Furthermore, it was suggested that severe injury to this "vulnerable" arm which would cause even greater pain and damage was about to occur. The "vulnerable" arm was then exposed on three spots blackened with India ink, to a standard noxious stimulation (500 mcal/cm²/sec for 3 sec.). In some of the experiments, after an interval of fifteen-thirty minutes during which hypnosis was continued, suggestions that the other arm was either "anaesthetic" or "normal" were repeated and reinforced. It was then similarly exposed on three spots to the standard noxious stimulation. To provide a control procedure, the order of exposing the "vulnerable" or "anaesthetic" arm to noxious stimulation was reversed. Also, the right arm was suggested to be "vulnerable" in some experiments, the left in others. In a number of the experiments, the suggestion of "vulnerability" for one arm and "anaesthesia" for the other were made simultaneously and the noxious stimulation was applied during the same interval alternately on the two arms.

The inflammatory reaction and tissue damage were assessed by observations and measurements of area, intensity and duration of erythema, edema, blister formation, necrosis and when present, residual scar formation. Photographs were made approximately twenty minutes after the end of an experiment, and at twenty-four-hour intervals for about two weeks. In almost all experiments, the inflammatory reaction and the subsequent evidence of tissue damage were greater on the side of suggested pain and vulnerability (Fig. 40). It was also evident that the effect of

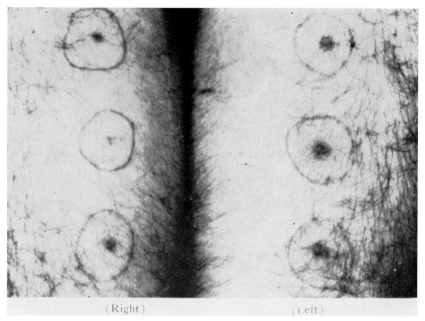

(Right)   (Left)

Figure 40. Photograph of the arms three days after noxious thermal stimulation during hypnosis. The burns were made in quick alternation from one arm to the other while the left was being suggested as "vulnerable," the right arm as "anaesthetic."

suggested "anaesthesia" was to suppress the inflammatory reaction as contrasted with no suggestion or suggestion of normality.

The explanation for the greater damage occurring in the arm suggested to be vulnerable when identical noxious stimulation had been delivered to both arms appeared to lie in the fact that a greater and longer sustained rise in the skin temperature was recorded in the "vulnerable" arm during hypnosis and following exposure to the damaging stimulus (Figs. 41 and 42).

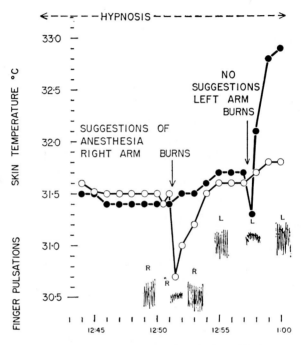

Figure 41. Measurements during hypnosis of the skin temperature and amplitude of finger pulsations of the right "anaesthetic" arm and of the left arm stated to be normally sensitive. Note the larger initial vaso-constriction as indicated by fall in skin temperature in the arm suggested to be anaesthetic (right), and the markedly reduced subsequent vasodilatation as compared to the reaction to the burns on the normally sensitive side (left). The absence of or the minimal vasodilatation after injury in the arm suggested to be "anaesthetic" affords a partial explanation of the minimal effect of injury.

The greater rise in skin temperature occurred in all experiments in which damage was greater on the "vulnerable" arm. A corresponding increase in finger pulsations was frequently seen, but could be less predictably measured.

Ely and associates produced inflammatory wheals in the fore-

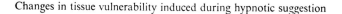

Changes in tissue vulnerability induced during hypnotic suggestion

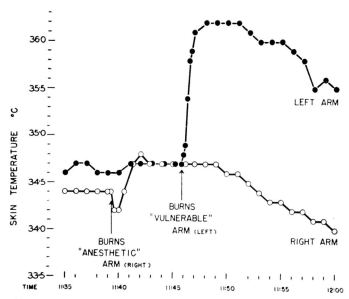

Figure 42. Measurements during hypnosis of the skin temperature of the right ("anaesthetic") and the left ("vulnerable") arm previous to, during and following the application of a damaging heat stimulus (500 mcal·cm^{-2}·sec^{-1} for 3 sec). The right arm was suggested to be numb, anaesthetic and without feeling, whereas the left arm was suggested to be already damaged, painful and about to be injured further. Note the greater degree and more persistent rise of skin temperature after suggestion of damage, indicating the pertinence of vasodilatation to the enhanced inflammatory reaction to injury.

arms of human subjects by injecting dilute trypsin solution. A relatively great inflammatory response was found to correlate with a low normal plasma concentration of corticosteroids (164).

Enhanced inflammation has been shown to be effective in combating invasion by micro-organisms and in the rapid elimination of tissue breakdown products of injury. The changes described in these experiments may indicate that man includes among his adaptive and protective devices, neural reactions integrated at the highest levels that heighten inflammation in the peripheral tissues and thus increase the local susceptibility to injury, at the same time enhancing the protection of the whole organism. Such adaptive reactions at times may be essential to survival. When evoked inappropriately or excessively, however, they may cause mildly damaging stimuli to result in relatively great injury and thus contribute to disease.

BIBLIOGRAPHY

1. WOLFF, H. G.: *Headache and Other Head Pain.* New York, Oxford, 1948 and 1963.
2. GRAHAM, J. R., and WOLFF, H. G.: Mechanism of migraine headache and action of ergotamine tartrate. *Proc. Ann. Res. Nerv. Ment. Dis., 18*:638-669, 1937. Also: *Arch. Neurol. Psychiat., 39*:737-763, 1938.
3. WOLFF, H. G.: Headache mechanism. Transactions, Collegium Internationale Allergologicum. *Int. Arch. Allerg.,* 7:210, 1955.
4. OSTFELD, A. M., CHAPMAN, L. F., GOODELL, H., and WOLFF, H. G.: Studies in headache. Summary of evidence concerning a noxious agent active locally during migraine headache. *Psychosom. Med., 19*:199-208, 1957.
5. CHAPMAN, L. F., RAMOS, A. O., GOODELL, H., SILVERMAN, G., and WOLFF, H. G.: A humoral agent implicated in vascular headache of the migraine type. *Arch Neurol., 3*:223, 229, 1960.
6. CHAPMAN, L. F., RAMOS, A. O., GOODELL, H., and WOLFF, H. G.: Neurokinin: A poly-peptide formed during neuronal activity in man. *Trans. Amer. Neurol. Ass.,* 1960, p. 42.
7. CHAPMAN, L. F., RAMOS, A. O., GOODELL, H., and WOLFF, H. G.: Neurohumoral features of afferent fibers in man. Their role in vasodilatation, inflammation and pain. *Arch. Neurol., 4*:617-650, 1961.
8. CHAPMAN, L. F., RAMOS, A. O., GOODELL, H., and WOLFF, H. G.: Evidence of Kinin Formation resulting from neural activity evoked by noxious stimulation. *Ann. N. Y. Acad. Sci., 104*:258-272, 1963.
9. WOLFF, H. G.: *Headache,* revised by H. Goodell, Lawrence E. Hinkle, Jr., and E. Charles Kunkle. In: *Signs and Symptoms.* C. M. MacBryde, Ed. Philadelphia, Lippincott, 1964, Chap. 4.
10. WOLFF, H. G.: The pathophysiology of headache (compiled from the writings of Harold G. Wolff, M.D., by Helen Goodell and Lawrence E. Hinkle, Jr.). *Int. J. Neurol., 3*:287-314, 1962.

11. DUNNING, H. S., Intracranial and extracranial vascular accidents in migraine. *Arch. Neurol. Psychiat.*, *48*:396, 1942.

12. OSTFELD, A. M., and WOLFF, H. G.: Studies on headache: Reactivity of bulbar conjunctival vessels during the migraine type of headache and muscle contraction headache. *Arch Neurol. Psychiat.*, *77*:113, 1957.

13. DALESSIO, D. J., CHAPMAN, L. F., ZILELI, T. CATTELL, M., EHRLICH, R., FORTUIN, F., GOODELL, H., and WOLFF, H. G.: Studies on headache. Responses of the bulbar conjunctival blood vessels during induced oliguria and diuresis and their modification by UML-491. *Arch Neurol.*, *5*:590-593, 1961.

14. PFEIFFER, J. B., and KUNKLE, E. C.: Fluctuations in cranial arterial tone as measured by "histamine responsiveness". *Trans. Amer. Neurol. Ass.*, *76*:244, 1951.

15. DALESSIO, D. J. CAMP, W. A., GOODELL, H., and WOLFF, H. G.: Studies on headache. The mode of action of UML-491 and its relevance to the nature of vascular headache of the migraine type. *Arch. Neurol.*, *4*:235-240, 1961. Also: *Trans. Amer. Neurol. Ass.*, 1961, pp. 95-98.

16. DALESSIO, D. J., CAMP, W. A., GOODELL, H., CHAPMAN, L. F., ZILELI, T., RAMOS, A. O., EHRLICH, R., FORTUIN, F., CATTELL, M., and WOLFF, H. G.: Studies on headache. The relevance of the prophylactic action of UML-491 in vascular headache of the migraine type to the pathophysiology of this syndrome. *World Neurol.*, *3*:66-71, 1962.

17. ZILELI, T., CHAPMAN, L. F., and WOLFF, H. G.: Anti-inflammatory action of UML-491 demonstrated by granuloma pouch technique in rats. *Arch. Int. Pharmacodyn.*, *136*:463, 1962.

18. GOODELL, H., LEWONTIN, R., and WOLFF, H. G.: Familial occurrence of migraine headache. A study of heredity. *Arch. Neurol. Psychiat.*, *72*:325-334, 1954.

19. WOLFF, H. G.: Personality features and reactions of patients with migraine. *Arch. Neurol. Psychiat.*, *37*:895-921, 1937.

20. MARCUSSEN, R. M., and WOLFF, H. G.: A formulation of the dynamics of the migraine attack. *Psychosom. Med.*, *11*:251-256, 1949.

21. SOURS, J. A., and ERDBRINK, W. L.: Psychophysiological false myopia: A parasympathetic depressive withdrawal reaction: Its differentiation from other psychogenic visual disturbances. *Aerospace Med.*, *35*:48-52, 1964.

22. DUKE-ELDER, SIR STEWART: *Text Book of Ophthalmology.* Vol. 5: *The Ocular Adnexa,* 5305. St. Louis, Mosby, 1952.

23. WOLF, S., and RIPLEY, H. S.: Reactions among allied prisoners of war subjected to three years of imprisonment and torture by the Japanese. *Amer. J. Psychiat., 104*:180, 1947.

24. WOLF, S., and MESSIER, P. E.: Corneal vascular changes in association with conflict in a patient with phlyctenular keratitis. *Proc. Ass. Res. Nerv. Ment. Dis., 29*:537, 1950.

25. LACQUEUR, L.: History of my glaucoma. The Sight Saving Review, Dec. 10, 1940. Trans. from *Klin. Augenhenk., 47*:639, 1909.

26. RIPLEY, H. S., and WOLFF, H. G.: Life situations, emotions and glaucoma. *Proc. Ass. Res. Nerv. Ment. Dis., 29*:523, 1950. Also: *Psychosom. Med., 12*:215-224, 1950.

27. HOLMES, T. H., GOODELL, H., WOLF, S., and WOLFF, H. G.: *The Nose: An Experimental Study of Reactions Within the Nose in Human Subjects.* Springfield, Thomas, 1950.

28. TENNYSON, A.: The Princess. Part 4, Song, Stanza I. *The Poems and Plays of Tennyson.* Modern Library Edition, New York, Random House, 1938.

29. HOLMES, T. H., TREUTING, T., and WOLFF, H. G.: Life situations, emotions and nasal disease: Evidence on summative effects exhibited in patients with hay fever. *Proc. Ann. Res. Nerv. Ment. Dis., 29*:545, 1950. Also: *Psychosom. Med., 13*:71, 1951.

30. GRACE, W. J., and GRAHAM, D. T.: The specificity of the relation between attitudes and disease. *Psychosom. Med., 14*: 243, 1952.

31. GRAHAM, D. T., LUNDY, R. M., BENJAMIN, L. S., KABLER, J. D., LEWIS, W. C., KUNISH, N. O., and GRAHAM, F. K.: Specific attitudes in initial interviews with patients having different "psychosomatic" diseases. *Psychosom. Med., 24*:257, 1962.

32. CANNON, W. B.: *Bodily Changes in Pain, Hunger, Fear and Rage.* New York, Appleton, 1929.

33. GROEN, J. J.,: *Psychosomatic Research.* London, Pergamon Press, 1964.

34. STEVENSON, I.: Variations in the secretion of bronchial mucus during periods of life stress. *Proc. Ass. Res. Nerv. Ment. Dis., 29*:596, 1950.

35. WOLF, G. A., and WOLFF, H. G.: Study on the nature of certain symptoms associated with cardiovascular disorders. *Psychosom. Med., 8*:293, 1946.

36. WOLF, S.: Sustained contraction of the diaphragm; the mechanism of a common type of dyspnea and precordial pain (Abstract). *J. Clin. Invest.*, *26*:1201, 1951.

37. EKLUND, G., VON EULER, C., and RUTKOWSKI, S.: Spontaneous and reflex activity of intercostal gamma motoneurones. *J. Physiol. (London)*, *171*:139-163, 1964.

38. FESSARD, ALBE, and SZABO, T.: Effects of variations in temperature on the activity of certain receptors of mormyridae. *C. R. Acad. Sci. (Paris)*, *254*:2084-5, 1962.

39. HINKLE, L. E., CHRISTENSON, W. N., KANE, F. D., OSTFELD, A., THETFORD, W. N., and WOLFF, H. G.: An investigation of the relation between life experience, personality characteristics, and general susceptibility to illness. *Psychosom. Med.*, *20*:278, 1958.

40. HINKLE, L. E., JR.: Ecological observations of the relation of physical illness, mental illness and the social environment. *Psychosom. Med.*, *23*:289, 1961.

41. HINKLE, L. E., JR., and CHRISTENSON, W. N.: Differences in amount of illness and in signs believed prognostic of atherosclerosis and hypertension in two groups of young men. *J.A.M.A.*, *177*:247, 1961 .

42. CHRISTENSON, WILLIAM N., BENJAMIN, BRY, KANE, F. D., PLUMMER, N., SCHAEFFER, M., WIDELOCK, D., and HINKLE, L. E., JR.: An outbreak of Asian Influenze in a closely observed group of women; Factors apparently influencing the clinical manifestations of illness. Presented to the Amer. Thoracic Society, Denver, May, 1963. Abst. *Amer. Rev. Resp. Dis.*, *88*:129, 1963.

43. BOGDONOFF, M. D., BOGDONOFF, M. M., and WOLF, S.: Studies on salivary function in man. Variations in secretory rates as part of the adaptive pattern. *J. Psychosom. Res.*, *5*:170-174, 1961.

44. WOLF, S.: Unpublished observations on halitosis.

45. WOLF, S., and ALMY, T. P.: Experimental observations on cardiospasm in man. *Gastroenterology*, *13*:401, 1949.

46. WOLF, S. G., and WOLFF, H. G.: *Human Gastric Function: An Experimental Study of a Man and His Stomach.* New York, Oxford, 1943 and 1947.

47. WOLF, S. G.: *The Stomach.* New York, Oxford, 1965.

48. MIRSKY, I. A.: Physiologic, psychologic and social determinants

in the etiology of duodenal ulcer. *Amer. J. Dig. Dis.* (New Series) *3(4)*:285-314, 1958.

49. WOLF, S.: Studies on nausea. Effects of ipecac and other emetics on the human stomach and duodenum. *Gastroenterology, 12*:212, 1949.

50. WOLF, S.: Observations on the occurrence of nausea among combat soldiers. *Gastroenterology, 8*:15, 1947.

51. GRACE, W. J., WOLF, S., and WOLFF, H. G.: *The Human Colon. An Experimental Study Based on Direct Observation of four fistulous subjects.* New York, Hoeber, 1951.

52. ARFWIDDSON, S.: Pathogenesis of multiple diverticula of the sigmoid colon in diverticular disease. *Acta Chir. Scand.* (Suppl) 342, 1964.

53. Almy, T.: The Physiology and Abnormal Physiology of the Colon. Read at May 27th meeting of American Gastroenterological Association, Montreal, 1965.

54. RANDALL, W. C., Ed: *Nervous Control of the Heart.* Baltimore, William and Wilkins, 1965.

55. McCLURE, C. M.: Cardiac arrest through volition. *Calif. Med., 90*:440, 1959.

56. GORDON, H. I., JR., WHALEN, R. E., and BOGDONOFF, M. D.: Heart rate changes in physicians during daily 'stressful' tasks. *J. Psychosom. Res., 7*:147-151, 1963.

57. SCHOLANDER, P. F.: Physiological adaptation to diving in animals and man. *Harvey Lect., 57*:93, 1961-62.

58. RICHTER, CURT P.: On the phenomenon of sudden death in animals and man. *Psychosom. Med., 19*:191-198, 1957.

59. WOLF, S.: Sudden death and the oxygen-conserving reflex. *Amer. Heart J., 71*:840, 1966.

60. WOLF, S., CARDON, P., SHEPARD, E., and WOLFF, H. G.: *Life Stress and Essential Hypertension.* Baltimore, Williams and Wilkins, 1955.

61. STEVENSON, I., and DUNCAN, C. H.: Alterations in cardiac function and circulatory efficiency during periods of life stress as shown by changes in the rate, rhythm, electrocardiographic pattern and output of the heart in those with cardiovascular disease. *Proc. Ass. Res. Nerv. Ment. Dis., 29*:799, 1950.

62. WOLF, STEWART: Cardiovascular reactions to symbolic stimuli. *Circulation, 18*:287-292, 1958.

63. DUNCAN, C. H., STEVENSON, I. P., and WOLFF, H. G.: Life situa-

tions, emotions and exercise tolerance. *Psychosom. Med.,* *13*:36, 1951.

64. Stevenson, I. P., Duncan, C. H., and Ripley, H. S.: Variations in the electrocardiogram with changes in emotional state. *Geriatrics, 6*:164, 1951.

65. Wolf, S.: Relative burdens of emotion and exercise on the cardiovascular system. In: *Work and the Heart.* New York, Hoeber, 1959.

66. Wasserburger, R. H., Siebecker, K. L., Jr., and Lewis, W. C.: Effect of hyperventilation on normal adult electrocardiogram. *Circulation, 13*:850, 1956.

67. Hinkle, L. E., Jr., Carver, S., Benjamin, B., Christenson, W. N., and Strong, B. W.: Studies in ecology of coronary heart disease. I. Variations in the human electrocardiogram under conditions of daily life. *Arch. Environ. Health* (Chicago), *9*:14-20, 1964.

68. Hellerstein, H. K.: Work load and cardiac function. In: *Conference on Heart in Industry.* New York Heart Association, 1959, p. 25.

69. Ford, A. B., and Hellerstein, H. K.: Energy expenditure by cardiac and non-cardiac workers. First Wisconsin Conference on Work and the Heart, Milwaukee, 1957.

70. Ford, A. B., and Hellerstein, H. K.: Work and heart disease. I. A physiologic study in the factory. *Circulation, 18*:823, 1958.

71. Ford, A. B., Hellerstein, H. K., and Turell, D.: Work and heart disease. II. A physiologic study in a steel mill. *Circulation, 20*:257, 1959.

72. Sarnoff, S. J., Braunwald, E., Welch, G. H., Jr., Case, R. B., Stainsby, W. N., and Marcuz, R.: Hemodynamic determinants of oxygen consumption of the heart with special reference to the tension-time index. *Amer. J. Physiol., 192*: 148, 1958.

73. Gerola, A., Feinberg, H., and Katz, L. N.: Oxygen cost of cardiac hemodynamic activity. *Physiologist, 1*:31, 1957.

74. Christenson, W. N., and Hinkle, L. E., Jr.; Differences in illness and prognostic signs in two groups of young men. *J.A.M.A., 177*:247-253 1961.

75. Hickam, J. B., Cargill, W. H., and Golden, A.: Cardiovascular reactions to emotional stimuli. Effect on the cardiac output, arteriovenous oxygen difference, arterial pressure, and peripheral resistance. *J. Clin. Invest., 27*:290, 1948.

76. Duncan, C. H., Stevenson, I. P., and Ripley, H. S.: Life situations, emotions and paroxysmal auricular arrhythmias. *Psychosom. Med., 12*:23, 1950.

77. Wolf, S.: Disease as a way of life. Neural integration in systemic pathology. *Perspect. Biol. Med.,* pp. 288-305, Spring, 1961.

78. Schneider, R. A.: The relation of stress to clotting time, relative viscosity and certain other biophysical alterations of the blood in the normotensive and hypertensive subjects. *Proc. Ass. Res. Nerv. Ment. Dis., 29*:818, 1950.

79. Wolf, S., Pfeiffer, J. B., Ripley, H. S., Winter, O. S., and Wolff, H. G.: Hypertension as a reaction pattern to stress: Summary of experimental data on variations in blood pressure and renal blood flow. *Ann. Intern. Med., 29*:1956, 1948.

80. Brod, J., French, V., Hejl, Z., and Zirka, J.: Circulatory changes underlying blood pressure elevation during acute emotional stress (mental arithmetic) in normotensive and hypertensive subjects. *Clin. Sci., 18*:269, 1959.

81. Alexander, F.: Emotional factors in essential hypertension. *Psychosom. Med., 1*:173, 1939.

82. Smithwick, R. H.: The effect of sympathectomy upon the mortality and survival rates of patients with hypertensive cardiovascular disease. In: *"Hypertension"*, E. T. Bell, Ed. Minneapolis, Univ. Minnesota Press, 1951, p. 429.

83. Seifter, J., Baeder, C., Zarafonetis, C., and Kalas, J.: Effect of adrenals, pituitary, liver and mucopolysaccharides on blood lipids. In: *Hormones and Atherosclerosis.* Proc. Conference in Brighton, Utah, 1958. G. Pincus, Ed. New York, Acad. Press, 1959.

84. Naughton, John, and Balke, Bruno: Physical working capacity in medical personnel and the response of serum cholesterol to acute exercise and to training. *Amer. J. Med. Sci., 247*:286-292, 1964.

85. Wolf, S., McCabe, W. R., Yamamoto, J., Adsett, C. A., and Schottstaedt, W. W.: Changes in serum lipid in relation to emotional stress during rigid control of diet and exercise. *Circulation, 26*:379-387, 1962.

86. Thomas, C. B., and Murphy, E. A.: Further studies on cholesterol levels in the Johns Hopkins Medical Students: Effect of stress at examinations. *J. Chronic Dis., 8*:661, 1958.

87. Wertlake, P. T., Wilcox, A. A., Haley, M. I., and Peterson,

J. E.: Relationship of mental and emotional stress to serum cholesterol levels. *Proc. Soc. Exp. Biol. Med., 97*:163, 1958.

88. GRUNDY, S. M., and GRIFFIN, A. C.: Effects of periodic mental stress on serum cholesterol levels. *Circulation, 19*:496, 1959.

89. DREYFUSS, F., and CZACKES, J. W.: Blood cholesterol and uric acid of healthy medical students under stress of an examination. *Arch. Int. Med., 103*:708, 1959.

90. GROEN, J. J., TIJONG, B. K., WILLEBRANDT, A. F., and KAMMINGA, C. J.: Influence of nutrition, individuality and different forms of stress on blood cholesterol: Results of an experiment of 9 months duration in 60 normal volunteers. Proc. First International Congress of Dietetics. Voeding, V. 10, 1959.

91. GROOVER, M. E., JR.: Clinical evaluation of a public health program to prevent coronary artery disease. *Trans. Coll. Physicians, 24*:105, Philadelphia, 1957.

92. FRIEDMAN, M., ROSENMAN, R. H., and CARROLL, V.: Changes in the serum cholesterol and blood clotting time in men subjected to cyclic variation of occupational stress. *Circulation, 17*:852, 1958.

93. HAMMARSTEN, J. F., CATHEY, C., REDMOND, R. F., and WOLF, S.: Serum cholesterol, diet and stress in patients with coronary artery disease. (Abstract). *J. Clin. Invest., 36*:897, 1957.

94. ADSETT, C. A., SCHOTTSTAEDT, W. W., and WOLF, S.: Changes in coronary blood flow and other hemodynamic indicators induced by stressful interviews. *Psychosom. Med., 24*:331-336, 1962.

95. BOGDONOFF, MORTON D. and ESTES, E. HARVEY, JR.: Energy dynamics and acute states of arousal in man. *Psychosom. Med., 23* (1) :23-32, 1961.

96. CARDON, P. V., JR., and GORDON, R. S., JR.: Rapid increase of plasma unesterified fatty acids in man during fear. *J. Psychosom. Res., 4*:5-9, 1959.

97. OLIVER, M. F., and BOYD, G. S.: Some current views on the aetiology of coronary artery disease (Symposium on Coronary Artery Disease). *Brit. Heart J., 19*:582, 1957.

98. RUSSEK, H. I., and ZOHMAN, B. L.: Relative significance of heredity, diet, and occupational stress in coronary heart disease of young adults: Based on an analysis of 100 patients between the ages of 25 and 40 years and a similar group of

100 normal control subjects. *Amer. J. Med. Sci.*, *235*:266, 1958.

99. DREYFUSS, F.: Role of emotional stress preceding coronary occlusion. *Amer. J. Cardiol.*, *3*:590, 1959.

100. WEISS, E., DLIN, B., ROLLIN, H. R., FISCHER, H. K., and BEPLER, C. R.: Emotional factors in coronary occlusion. I. Introduction and general summary. *Arch Int. Med.*, *99*:628, 1957.

101. SCHNEIDER, ROBERT A., and COSTILOE, J. PAUL: Relationship of sinus arrhythmia to age and its prognostic significance in ischemic heart disease. *Clin. Res.*, *13(2)*:219, 1965 (Abstract).

102. HAMPTON, J. W., MANTOOTH, J., BRANDT, E. N., and WOLF, S.: Plasma fibrinogen patterns in patients with coronary atherosclerosis *Circulation*, *34*:1098, 1966.

103. SCHOTTSTAEDT, W. W., BRUHN, JOHN, G., and ADSETT, ALEX: Unpublished data.

104. SCHOTTSTAEDT, W. W., GRACE, W. J., and WOLFF, H. G.: Life situations, behavior patterns, and renal excretion of fluid and electrolytes. *J.A.M.A.*, *157*:1485-1488, 1955.

105. PFEIFFER, J. B., JR., and WOLFF, H. G.: Studies in renal circulation during periods of life stress and accompanying emotional reactions in subjects with and without essential hypertension: Observations on the role of neural activity in regulation of renal blood flow. *Proc. Ass. Res. Nerv. Ment. Dis.*, *29*:929, 1950. Also: *J. Clin. Invest.*, *29*:1227, 1950.

106. SCHOTTSTAEDT, W. W., GRACE, WILLIAM, J., and WOLFF, H. G.: Life situations, behavior, attitudes, emotions and renal excretion of fluid and electrolytes. I. Method of study. *J. Psychosom. Res.*, *1*:75-83, 1956.

107. SCHOTTSTAEDT, W. W., GRACE, WILLIAM J., and WOLFF, H. G.: Life situations, behavior, attitudes, emotions and renal excretion of fluid and electrolytes. II. Retention of water and sodium. *J. Psychosom. Res.*, *1*:147-159, 1956.

108. SCHOTTSTAEDT, W. W., GRACE, WILLIAM J., and WOLFF, H. G.: Life situations, behavior, attitudes, emotions and renal excretion of fluid and electrolytes. III. Diuresis of fluid and electrolytes. *J. Psychosom. Res.*, *1*:203-211, 1956.

109. SCHOTTSTAEDT, W. W., GRACE, WILLIAM J., and WOLFF, H. G.: Life situations, behavior, attitudes, emotions and renal excretion of fluid and electrolytes. IV. Situations associated with retention of water, sodium and potassium, *Trans. Ass. Amer. Physicians.*, *70*:158, 1957.

110. LUETSCHER, JOHN A., and LIEBERMAN, AMOS H.: Idiopathic edema with increased aldosterone output. *Trans. Ass. Amer. Physicians, 70*:158, 1957.

111. STRAUB, L. R., RIPLEY, H. S., and WOLF, STEWART: Disturbances in bladder function in association with varying life situations and emotional stress. *J.A.M.A., 141*:1139, 1949.

112. WOLF, S.: Disorders of bladder function. In: *The Psychological Basis of Medical Practice*, Harold Lief, Victor F. Lief and Nina R. Lief, Eds. New York, Hoeber, 1963, Chap. 28, p. 339.

113. RIPLEY, H. S., and WOLF, S.: Unpublished observations on patient E. G. and others.

114. McLELLAN, ALLISTER M., and GOODELL, HELEN: Pain from the bladder, ureter and kidney pelvis. *Proc. Ass. Res. Nerv. Ment. Dis., 23*:252, 1943.

115. WOLF, S., and RIPLEY, H. S.: Studies on the action of intravenously administered sodium amytal. *Amer. J. Med. Sci., 215*:56, 1948.

116. WOLF, S.: Emotions and disease. *Physiology for Physicians.* Vol. 1, No. 2, February, 1963.

117. STRAUB, LEONARD R., RIPLEY, H. S., and WOLF, STEWART: An experimental approach to psychosomatic bladder disorders. *New York J. Med., 49*:635, 1949.

118. ASSALI, N.: Toxemias of pregnancy. *Heart Bull., 11*:36-39, 1962.

119. MANN, EDWARD C.: Psychiatric investigation of habitual abortion. *Obstet. Gynec., 7*:589-601, 1956.

120. MANN, EDWARD C.: Habitual abortion. *Amer. J. Obstet. Gynec., 77*:706-718, 1959.

121. MANN, EDWARD C.: Emotional reactions occurring in relation to obstetrical complications. *Conference Papers of the Chicago Medical Society,* January, 1960, pp. 127-131.

122. DUNCAN, CHARLES H., and TAYLOR, HOWARD C. JR.: A psychosomatic study of pelvic congestion. *Amer. J. Obstet. Gynec., 64*:1, 1952.

123. STRAUB, LEONARD, and WOLF, S.: Unpublished observations.

124. TAYLOR, HOWARD C.: Vascular congestion and hyperemia. *Amer. J. Obstet. Gynec., 57*:211, 1949.

125. HINKLE, L. E., JR., CONGER, G. B., and WOLF, S.: Studies on diabetes mellitus: The relation of stressful life situations to the concentration of ketone bodies in the blood of diabetic and non-diabetic humans. *J. Clin. Invest., 29*:754, 1950.

126. HINKLE, L. E., JR., EDWARDS, C. J., and WOLF, S.: Occurrence of diuresis in humans in stressful situations and its possible relation to the diuresis of early starvation. *J. Clin. Invest.*, *30*:809, 1951.

127. HINKLE, L. E., JR., EDWARDS, C. J., and WOLF, S.: Studies in diabetes Mellitus. II. Occurence of a diuresis in diabetic persons exposed to stressful life situations with experimental observations on its relation to the concentration of glucose in blood and urine. *J. Clin. Invest.*, *30*:818, 1951.

128. HINKLE, L. E., JR., EVANS, F. M., and WOLF, S.: Studies in diabetes mellitus. III. Life history of three labile diabetics and relation of significant experiences in their lives to the onset and course of the disease. *Psychosom. Med.*, *13*:160, 1951.

129. HINKLE, L. E., JR., EVANS, F. M., and WOLF, STEWART (with technical assistance of G. Conger, C. J. Edwards and Betty Pugh): Studies in diabetes mellitus. IV. Life history of three persons with relatively mild, stable diabetes and relation of significant experiences in their lives to the onset and course of disease. *Psychosom. Med.*, *13*:184, 1951.

130. HINKLE, L. E., JR. and WOLF, S.: Experimental study of life situations, emotions and the occurrence of acidosis in a Jew. *Amer. J. Med. Sci.*, *217*:130, 1949.

131. WOLFF, H. G., TUNIS, M. M., and GOODELL, H.: Evidence of tissue damage and changes in pain sensitivity in subjects with vascular headaches of the migraine type. *Arch. Intern. Med. (Chicago)*, *92*:478, 1953.

132. HETZEL, BASIL S., GRACE, W. J., and WOLFF, H. G.: General metabolic changes during stressful life experience. *J. Psychosom. Res.*, *1*:186-202, 1956.

133. HETZEL, BASIL S.: Thyroid secretion in health and disease. *Aust. Ann. Med.*, *13*:80, 1964.

134. BROWN, L. B., HETZEL, and BASIL, S.: Stress, personality and thyroid disease. *J. Psychosom. Res.*, *7*:223, 1963.

135. FALCONER, I. R., and HETZEL, B. S.: The effect of emotional stress and TSH on thyroid vein hormone level in the exteriorised sheep thyroid. *Endocrinology*, 75:42, 1964.

136. LIDZ, THEODORE: Emotional factors in the etiology of hyperthyroidism. *Psychosom. Med.*, *11*:2, 1949.

137. GREILAND, R.: Thyrotozicosis at Ulleval Hospital in the years 1934-1944 with a special view to frequency of the disease. *Acta. Med. Scand.*, *125*:108, 1946.

138. SELYE, H.: *The Physiology and Pathology of Exposure in Stress.* Montreal, Acta, Inc., 1950.

139. HETZEL, B., SCHOTTSTAEDT, W. W., GRACE, W. J. and WOLFF, H. G.: Changes in urinary 17-hydroxycorticosteroid excretion during stressful life experiences in man. *J. Clin. Endocrinol., 10*:57, 1955.

140. SHENKIN, HENRY A.: The effect of pain on the diurnal pattern of plasma corticoid levels. *Neurology, 14*:1112, 1964.

141. LEVI, LENNART: The urinary output of adrenalin and noradren· alin during pleasant and unpleasant emotional states. *Psychosom. Med., 27*:80, 1965.

142. RAHMAN, L., RICHARDSON, H. B., and RIPLEY, H. S.: Anorexia nervosa with psychiatric observations. *Psychosom. Med., 1*:335· 365, 1939.

143. BLISS, EUGENE L., and BRANCH, C. H. HARDIN: *Anorexia Nervosa. Its History, Psychology and Biology.* New York, Hoeber, 1960.

144. STUNKARD, A. J., and WOLFF, H. G.: Pathogenesis in human obesity. Function and disorder of a mechanism of satiety. *Psychosom. Med., 20*:17-29, 1958.

145. MILLER, N. E.: Shortcomings of food consumption as a measure of hunger; results from other behavioral techniques. *Ann. N. Y. Acad. Sci., 63*:141, 1955.

146. STUNKARD, A. J., GRACE, W. J., and WOLFF, H. G.: The night eating syndrome. A pattern of food intake among certain obese patients. *Amer. J. Med., 19*:78-86, 1955.

147. STUNKARD, A. J.: The dieting depression. Incidence and clinical characteristics of untoward responses to weight reduction regimens. *Amer. J. Med., 23*:77-86, 1957.

148. GOLDBLATT, P. B., MOORE, M. E., and STUNKARD, A. J.: Social factors in obesity. *J.A.M.A., 192*:1039-1044, 1965.

149. BARKER, W., and BARKER, S.: Experimental production of human convulsive brain potentials by stress induced effects upon neural integrative function: Dynamics of the convulsive reaction to stress. *Proc. Ass. Res. Nerv. Ment. Dis., 29*:90, 1950.

150. BARKER, WAYNE: Studies in epilepsy: Personality pattern, situational stress and the symptoms of narcolepsy. *Psychosom. Med., 10*:193, 1948.

151. BARKER, WAYNE, and WOLF, STEWART: Experimental induction of Grand Mal seizure during the hypnoidal state induced by Sodium Amytal. *Amer. J. Med Sci., 214*:600, 1947.

152. WOLF, S: Observation during World War II. Unpublished.
153. GRAHAM, D. T., and GOODELL, H., and WOLFF, H. G.: Neural mechanisms involved in itch, "itchy skin" and "tickle sensations. *J. Clin. Invest.*, *30*:37-49, 1951.
154. GRAHAM, D. T., GOODELL, H., and WOLFF, H. G.: Studies on pain. The relation between cutaneous vasodilatation, pain threshold and spontaneous itching and pain. *Amer. J. Med. Sci.*, *234*:420-430, 1957.
155. GRAHAM, D. T.: The pathogenesis of hives: Experimental study of life situations, emotions and cutaneous vascular reactions. *Proc. Ass. Res. Nerv. Ment. Dis.*, *29*:987, 1950.
156. GRAHAM, D. T., and WOLF, STEWART: The pathogenesis of urticaria. Experimental study of life situations, emotions, and cutaneous vascular reactions. *J.A.M.A.*, *143*:1396, 1950.
157. DI PALMA, J. R., REYNOLDS, S. R. M., and FOSTER, F. S.: Quantitative measurement of reactive hypermia in human skin. *Amer. Heart J.*, *23*:377, 1942.
158. GRAHAM, D. T., and WOLF, S.: The relation of eczema to attitude and to vascular reactions of the human skin. *J. Lab. Clin. Med.*, *42*:238, 1953.
159. LORENZ, THOMAS H., GRAHAM, D. T., and WOLFF, H. G.: A method for the collection and quantitative determination of sebum: Its application to an investigation of human sebum secretion. *J. Lab. Clin. Med.*, *39*:91-104, 1952.
160. WOLFF, H. G., LORENZ, T. H., and GRAHAM, D. T.: Stress, emotions and human sebum: Their relevance to acne vulgaris. *Trans. Ass. Amer. Physicians*, *64*:435, 1951.
161. WOLFF, H. G.: Disease and patterns of behavior. In: *The Hour of Insight: Sequel to Moments of Personal Discovery from Religion and Civilization Series*, R. M. McIver, Ed. New York, Harper, 1953, pp. 29-39. Also see: *Patients, Physicians and Illness*. E. Garthy Jaco, Ed. Chicago, Free Press, 1958, pp. 54-60.
162. BILISOLY, F. N., GOODELL, H., and WOLFF, H. G.: Vasodilatation, lowered pain threshold, and increased tissue vulnerability. Effects dependent upon peripheral nerve function. *Arch. Intern. Med. (Chicago)*, *94*:759-773, 1954.
163. CHAPMAN, L. F., GOODELL, H., and WOLFF, H. G.: Augmentation of the inflammatory reaction by activity of the central nervous system. *Arch. Neurol.*, *1*:557-582, 1959.

164. ELY, N. E., VERHEY, J. W., and HOLMES, T. H.: Experimental studies of skin inflammation. *Psychosom. Med., 25*:264, 1963.

165. WARDWELL, WALTER I., BAHNSON, CLAUS B. and CARON, HERBERT S.: Social and psychological factors in coronary heart disease. *J. Health and Human Behavior, 4*:154-165, 1963.

166. SYME, S. LEONARD, HYMAN, MERTON M. and ENTERLINE, P. E.: Cultural mobility and the occurrence of coronary heart disease. *J. Health and Human Behavior, 6*:178-189, 1965.

167. WELMER, A. and GROEN, J. J.: Effect of a simple deconditioning procedure on the diuretic and natriuretic response to a hypertonic salt load of hypertensive patients. (In press.)

168. EULER, U. S. v., GEMZELL, C. A., LEVI, L. and STROM, G.: Cortical and medullary adrenal activity in emotional stress. *Acta endocinol., 30*:567, 1959.

169. HARVEY, W. PROCTOR and LEVINE, SAMUEL A.: Paroxysmal ventricular tachycardia due to emotion. *J.A.M.A., 150*:479, 1952.

ADDITIONAL BIBLIOGRAPHY

1. ALEXANDER, FRANZ and FRENCH, THOMAS M.: *Psychoanalytic Therapy. Principles and Application.* New York, The Ronald Press Company, 1946.

2. ALEXANDER, FRANZ: *Psychosomatic Medicine, Its Principles and Applications.* New York, W. W. Norton and Co., 1950.

3. BYKOV, K. M. (Translated by W. Horsley Gantt): *The Cerebral Cortex and the Internal Organs.* New York, The Chemical Publishing Co., 1957.

4. CARBALLO, J. ROF: *Urdimbre Afectiva y Enfermedad.* Editorial Labor, S.A., 1961.

5. DUNBAR, FLANDERS: *Emotions and Bodily Changes,* 2nd Ed. A Survey of Literature on Psychosomatic Interrelationships, 1910-1933. New York, Columbia University Press, 1938.

6. DUNBAR, FLANDERS: *Psychiatry in the Medical Specialties.* New York, McGraw-Hill Book Co., Inc., 1959.

7. ENGEL, GEORGE: *Psychological Development in Health and Disease.* Philadelphia, W. B. Saunders Company, 1962.

8. GELLHORN, ERNST and LOOFBOURROW, G. N.: *Emotions and Emotional Disorders.* A Neurophysiological Study. New York, Harper and Row, 1963.

8a. GELLHORN, ERNST: *Principles of Autonomic-Somatic Integrations*

—*Physiological Basis of Psychological and Clinical Implica-tions.* Minneapolis, Univ. of Minnesota Press, 1967.

9. GREENFIELD, NORMAN S. and LEWIS, WILLIAM C. (Eds.) : *Psycho-analysis and Current Biological Thoughts.* Madison, Wisc., University of Wisconsin Press, 1965.

10. GRINKER, R.: *Psychosomatic Research.* New York, W. W. Norton Co., Inc., 1953.

11. GRINKER, ROY R. and ROBBINS, FRED P.: *Psychosomatic Case Book.* New York, The Blakiston Co., Inc., 1954.

12. HAMILTON, MAX: *Psychosomatics.* London, Chapman and Hall, 1955.

12a. JANIS, IRVING L.: *Psychological Stress.* New York, John Wiley and Sons, Inc., 1958.

13. KNUTSON, ANDRE L.: *The Individual Society and Health Be-havior.* New York, Russell Sage Foundation, 1965.

13a. LANGNER, THOMAS S. and MICHAEL, STANLEY I.: *Life Stress and Mental Health.* The Midtown Manhattan Study. London, The Macmillan Co., 1963.

14. NODINE, JOHN H. and MOYER, JOHN H. (Eds.) : *Psychosomatic Medicine—The First Hahnemann Symposium.* Philadelphia, Lea and Febiger, 1962.

14a. RAAB, WILHELM (Ed.) : *Ischemic Heart Disease.* Springfield, Ill., Thomas, 1966.

15. SCHOTTSTAEDT, WILLIAM W.: *Psychophysiologic Approach in Medical Practice.* Chicago, The Year Book Publishers, Inc., 1960.

16. SEGUIN, C. ALBERTO: *Introduction a la Medicina Psicosomatica.* Lima, Peru, Emp. Grafica T Scheuch S.A., 1947.

17. SIMON, A., HERBERT, C. C., STRAUSS, R. (Eds.) : *The Physiology of Emotions.* Springfield, Ill., Thomas, 1961.

17a. SPARER, PHINEAS J. (Ed.) : *Personality, Stress and Tuberculosis.* New York, International Universities Press, 1956.

18. WITMER, HELEN L. (Ed.) : *Teaching Psychotherapeutic Medicine.* New York, The Commonwealth Fund, 1947.

19. WITTKOWER, ERIC D. and CLEGHORN, R. A. (Eds.) : *Recent Devel-opments in Psychosomatic Medicine.* Philadelphia, J. B. Lip-pincott Company, 1954.

20. WORLD FEDERATION OF MENTAL HEALTH: *Uprooting and Resettle-ment.* New York, World Federation for Mental Health, 1960.

Chapter IV

THE ORGANIZATION OF REACTION PATTERNS

D<small>URING THE LAST QUARTER</small> of the nineteenth century, it became increasingly apparent to physiologists studying the functions of a single organ that they had to take into account the host of bodily responses that occurred when unanesthetized and intact experimental animals were injured by preparation for the test procedure. Also, the responses of animals which apparently were experiencing pain often were indistinguishable from the behavior of frightened animals who were neither injured nor in pain. Physiologists at last had to face the fact that regardless of what functions might be exhibited in an isolated organ, in the intact animal all functions are influenced by central integrative action.

Responses of the organism to destructive or painful stimulation and to circumstances perceived as threatening were seen by some physiologists as a fragmented, scattered and meaningless jumble, as the product of the spread of excitation because of anatomic contiguity within the nervous system, or as the haphazard effects of circulating chemical agents. Yet, these reactions do not fit into any simple structural, chemical, or mechanistic system. For example, in any one such reaction, all parts of the gastrointestinal system are not involved, nor is the entire cardiovascular or ventilatory system implicated in any one response. Moreover, skeletal muscle reactions may be linked with gastrointestinal and cardiovascular responses. In a given response, different anatomic divisions of the nervous system may be simultaneously implicated.

When, in addition, what a person says and does are observed and recorded, it is hard to avoid the inference that these reactions in circumstances perceived as threatening, involving disparate systems, and parts, *are goal-directed responses,* and that they are the products of integration and featured by selection, arrangement and organization.

Furthermore, such reactions evoked during circumstances perceived as threatening are quite different when the threat has one significance rather than another. For example, as already described in the case of the human stomach, opposite patterns of reaction occur when, on the one hand, circumstances are perceived as terrifying, or, at the other extreme when a threat provokes aggressive action and violent anger. Readily recognizable are two extremes. Between these occur a gamut of responses featured by underactivity and overactivity. Each pattern is linked with definable features of behavior, attitudes and feelings.

THE CONCEPTS OF PURPOSE

Santayana once said that those who cannot remember the past are condemned to repeat it (1). Hence, the evolution of some of the assumptions of science is pertinent to this discussion. In the eighteenth century, Cullen, Pinel, Baglivi and others held that disorders of the nervous system underlie most disease processes. This emphasis dominated French concepts of disease in the first half of the nineteenth century. But, in the latter half of the century, the enthusiastic interest in part phenomena, abetted by the widespread use of the microscope in studying cellular alterations, overshadowed the earlier interest in generalized reactions, not only in France but throughout the world of scientific medicine.

Physical scientists, especially in the late nineteenth century and early part of the twentieth, avoided teleological interpretation, the concept that purpose was a factor in biological organization. The very word teleology was used only in derogation. Its long association with belief in a universe focused on man as the special favorite of a "Divine Creator" in whom resided "purpose" and "final cause" made teleology an unusable word and concept for physical science. The why of phenomena was waived while the what and how were vigorously pursued.

Furthermore, physics and chemistry became the models for

scientific method, whose validity was assumed to rest on precise measurement. The successes, the prestige of the methods, and the attitudes of the physical scientists so influenced the direction of thought that their methods were eagerly applied by biologists in the investigation of living systems. This orientation was often productive, as, for example, in the study by physiologists of salt and water metabolism (2).

But scholarly physicians, too, took physics and chemistry as the models for clinical science. Mindful of the hard-won battle necessary to establish in their discipline the experimental method and attitude as exemplified by physics, and proud of the extraordinary triumphs that had ensued, they were loath to trust data about total behavior derived from unstructured studies with many variables. They were even more loath to participate in such studies. Thus, the assumption grew among clinical investigators that for the study of man in his context, the scientific method was unsuitable.

With the beginning of the twentieth century, some perceptive scientists outside the discipline of medicine became discontented with the restrictions and increasing number of inconsistencies that confronted them and challenged the validity of their assumptions. Some pertinent quotations from mathematicians and physical scientists exemplify this change. Thus, according to Whitehead (3): "It cannot be too clearly understood that the various physical laws which appear to apply to the behavior of atoms are not mutually consistent as at present formulated. The appeal to mechanism on behalf of biology was in its origin an appeal to the well-attested self-consistent physical concepts expressing the basis of natural phenomena. But at present there is no such system of concepts." According to Woodger (4): "Biologists are apt to take a far too naive attitude towards physics, interpreting it more realistically and dogmatically than physicists themselves, without any understanding of its history, of its metaphysical basis or of the traditional difficulties which have been inherent in some of its concepts from the beginning. But, as everyone should know, these difficulties have become particularly acute at the present day and are the subject of much renewed controversy."

Now, Western medicine has survived several shifts of emphasis. For at least three or four centuries it has had differing insights and preferred kinds of knowledge, evident in the swing of interest from the whole man to the part, and then to the whole again. Thus, in the late sixteenth and seventeenth centuries there flourished intensive interest in part phenomena as expressed in the biochemical and biophysical schools of medicine, known respectively as iatro-chemical and iatro-physical.

Such preferred research and experiment brought with it even then the danger of separating the physician from the bedside of the patient. Some of the leaders in investigation and formulation actually practiced little medicine, if any. Further attempts were made to erect a complete structure of medicine upon philosophical and mathematical foundations.

The formulation of new theories and hypotheses by these teachers turned the attention of the physician away from an interest in and care of the sick. It certainly separated investigators from clinicians. Able persons having abandoned the study of patients, medical practice descended to little better than magic and incantations.

Fortunately, in the late eighteenth century, clinical medicine was rescued by the rise of a new interest in the whole patient and in the incredibly exact descriptions of diseases many of which have not been surpassed even to this day. But in the nineteenth century, interest again drifted away from the bedside, so that by the latter half of the century the study of parts and elements once more almost entirely consumed the interest and energies of creative minds.

Yet ironically, like the bringing of coals to Newcastle, the significance of a concept of biologic organizations was brought home indirectly through theoretical physics. For example, Eddington said, "We often think that when we have completed our study of one we know all about two, because two is one and one. We forget that we have still to make a study of *and*. Secondary physics is the study of *and*—that is to say, of organization" (5).

At the same time, a growing restiveness with the study of part phenomena led biologists once again to turn their interest toward the meaning of separate functions to the purposes of the entire creature. For example, the biochemist Krebs said, "The properties of living matter can never be fully explored and truly understood without making reference to some ends which they serve" (6), a view shared by J. B. S. Haldane (7) and Walter B. Cannon (8). Thus when biologists resumed the study of the form and function of parts of living systems in relation to the goals of the whole organism, biology once again became the science of life (9).

CROSS PURPOSES IN BEHAVIOR

Naturalists, and more particularly zoologists, attempting to understand the behavior of living creatures, by preference and training observe them in their context while laboratory experimenters divide phenomena into small sections of space and time. Thus naturalists are able to observe the course of life on a big scale.

Looking at living creatures in their environment, naturalists have discerned not only their purposive patterns of behavior but also what have been called displacement patterns, the performance of a biologically inappropriate action when an appropriate one is blocked. The behavior does not serve directly the survival of the individual or the species. Biologically, it is irrelevant to the situation in which it is performed. For example, a wild rat that is feeding, when disturbed by another rat of a different species, makes aggressive noises and motions toward the interloper. The latter flees. But the first rat, instead of immediately resuming feeding, starts to groom its face with its forepaws, an action which it would not ordinarily perform in the middle of feeding. Deprived of the object of its aggression, the rat resorts to an alternative and inappropriate behavior pattern (10, 11).

Another example: if an animal has the choice of two conflicting patterns of action, it may reject these both for one that is inappropriate. A herring gull, in a situation calling for either attack or running away, neither of which it can carry out, may resort to grass pulling, part of a nest-building pattern which is completely inappropriate to the circumstances. Or, a third example: gulls have been studied during the period of sitting on their eggs. If one egg is removed from the nest, the gull starts completely inappropriate nest-building movements. When more eggs are removed, the nest-building movements increase, and the number of such movements in a given time increase in proportion to the number of eggs removed. When all the eggs are removed, preening increases markedly (12). This indicates that displacement behavior may be expressed quantitatively.

Instances of such carefully studied patterns are now numerous but one more example showing displacement behavior in a fish as the outlet of the conflicting drives of attack and escape is pertinent. Male sticklebacks, as part of their sexual activities, dig pits into which females deposit their eggs. The pits are dug by head-down attacks and diving movements. These functions are executed within well-defined territories. Within its territory, a male stickleback attacks every other male. Outside its territory, the same male does not fight but flees before a stranger. But, when male sticklebacks meet at the boundary between their territories, they adopt head-down attitudes and diving movements pertinent to pit digging and do under such circumstances dig numerous holes. If male sticklebacks are forced to nest closely together, they dig almost continuously, resulting in a much pockmarked area or even one huge pit (13).

There is a rich variety of displaced adaptive patterns exhibited by man under multiple conditions of duress, incongruous behavior in a mortal crisis or holocaust, facial contortions and other tics in association with social embarrassment or the need to repress violent retaliation, vasomotor alterations as in blushing or blanching, and a host of alterations in visceral behavior discussed in the previous chapter.

FAULTY ADAPTATION AND THE USE OF COMPENSATORY MEASURES

When an individual feels himself to be seriously threatened and blocked in the pursuit or the attainment of his goals, his failure to achieve adaptation may be manifest in an uneasy feeling, usually ill-defined, which is best described as anxiety. The person may also have a sense of malaise and his thinking may not be clear.

Such anxiety is at least transiently experienced by everyone often without awareness of its basis, since an individual does not necessarily recognize all of his goals, and since the goals themselves are often in conflict. Anxiety may be mitigated when protective, defensive, and compensatory reactions are called into play, thus helping him through periods of great environmental demands.

A multitude of such protective devices may be set up even in the absence of awareness of anxiety. Unacceptable facts, situations, or conflicts may be repressed, forgotten, denied, misrepresented, pretended to be other than they are, made light of, joked or clowned about. Excessive attention and show of affection may be demanded. The pursuit of popularity may be overdone. Blame may be fixed on something outside oneself. Alibis and excuses may be used. A substitute for the insoluble conflict or circumstances may be attacked, overcome, resolved; or vicarious "success" may be achieved where perfectionism or tireless application can achieve results. A detached, impersonal, aloof, remote attitude may be assumed. The dilemma may be depersonalized, or the individual may withdraw from the struggle and become apathetic. He may substitute a pattern of reaction suitable for one purpose to meet a situation in which it is entirely ineffective.

Even those ominous reactions that feature the behavior of people with schizophrenia-depersonalization, or feeling and acting as though the catastrophe one faces is of no personal significance— even those can be used transiently as protective measures. Some Jewish internees on entering Nazi concentration camps with their families were confronted by the fact that, within minutes of separation from them, their wives, children, and parents had been murdered. Yet by depersonalizing this information they were able to remain organized and effective, adapting themselves to their assignments as laborers or professional workers (14).

FUNCTION OF ORGANS AND INTEGRITY OF TISSUE

Should the load become too great or the frustration too prolonged or profound, or should time fail to resolve a dilemma, defenses may break down and among other untoward effects allow an uneasy, tense, anxious mood to emerge. Primitive devices may then be called forth to supplement the first defense, and may continue to operate even though they are not completely effective. Behavior patterns involving alimentation or those with urinary, sexual, respiratory, ventilatory, cardiovascular, glandular, secretory, and vasomotor activity are common. These substitutions or displaced patterns—suggestive of those described earlier in the rat, gull and fish can function excessively and for long periods while the subject is otherwise relatively effective and free of the costly feelings of anxiety, tension, hostility and depression. Thus, the existence of illness may serve its own adaptive function (15-21). Were it not for the untoward effect on the bodily tissues themselves, such adaptive arrangements might go on indefinitely. Occasionally, as in neurocirculatory asthenia for example, an illness can persist without serious consequences to the body. But often, as in hypertension, irreversible tissue damage may result.

ANATOMICAL CHANGES IN RATS

A most dramatic demonstration of tissue changes occurring as the result of environmental pressures and stresses is seen in the "domestication" of rats, so carefully investigated by Richter (22).

Outstanding in the domesticated wild rat as compared to his undomesticated cousins, are the reduction in size of the adrenal and thyroid, and the increase in size of the pituitary glands; the augmented capacity to adjust to changes in food, to meet laboratory circumstances, including man, and to withstand stress without attacking neighboring animals. The process of domestication has evidently involved extraordinary adaptive changes in the rat (23-25). An extreme reaction to captivity is a reluctance to breed, and cannibalism, as manifested in the eating of those young that may be produced.

Selye (26) demonstrated inverse changes in laboratory-bred rats. Adrenal glands enlarged during adaptation to a variety of stresses, assaults and threats. Moreover, these structural changes were achieved in a relatively short time. A further basic contribution of these studies was the demonstration that in addition to changes in endocrine structure there were many parenchymal changes in other organs and tissues, notably vascular structures. Such alterations were in no way specific responses to the nature of the traumatizing agent or procedure.

PATTERNING OF BODILY CHANGES IN MAN

The investigations on man reported herewith show how radically form and function of structures may change not only during long standing, but even during amazingly brief periods of adverse circumstances. The question of "organ selection" is intriguing but still incompletely answered. That is, how does an organ become implicated in a biologic pattern of offense or defense (15)?

It seems likely that some dominant, deeply ingrained, protective reaction patterns in man may be stockbound, analogous to the retriever patterns in dogs, running pattern in horses, hoarding in squirrels, building and space orientation in birds and insects and sham death in the opossum. The implication is that the individual and his clan meet life in a particular way different from the members of other stocks. An individual may have been a potential "nose reactor" or "colon reactor" all his life without ever actually having called upon a particular protective pattern for sustained periods because he did not need to. A given protective pattern may remain inconspicuous during long periods of relative security, and then with stress, becomes evident as a disorder involving the gut, the heart and vascular system, the naso-respiratory apparatus, the skin or general metabolism.

That certain stocks possess proclivities, often indefinitely latent for the development of specific disorders, is strikingly illuminated by the observations of Flynn (27) and Sheldon and Ball (28) made on girl twins aged twenty. These girls, identical as far as could be ascertained from birth history, early photographs, dominant handedness, finger prints, palm prints, blood groups, somato-types, hair structure, and skeletal structures by x-ray, nevertheless exhibited important differences. One had had arterial hypertension for about eight years, the other was normotensive. One of the pair at birth, during infancy, through childhood, adolescence and young maturity was "behind" the other. Lighter in weight at birth, somewhat slower in growth, less well developed, burdened with more frequent and severe infections, less outgiving emotionally, less able to learn, less capable of evoking love, less imaginative in work and less hopeful of success in pursuit of a mate, she had been since infancy, in relation to her sister, in a position of an "also ran." It was this relatively lesser one who had developed the hypertension. Flynn was able to show that both girls reacted vigoriously as regards pressor and other cardiovascular hyperdynamic reactions in response to plunging their extremities in ice water. Also, as regards blood pressure elevation, both responded vigorously, though not to the same degree, during interviews in which pertinent personal data were brought into focus. It thus appears that not only were they "poured out of the same mold" as to their structure, but they responded similarly during stress. They exhibited identical protective patterns having to do with mobilization for action. Notwithstanding, only one had felt obliged to strive almost continuously from birth. It may be that the difference between the hypertensive and the normotensive is one of congenital defect, but it is hardly likely to be specific in terms of deranged blood pressure regulating apparatus. It is simpler to postulate that the hypertensive girl exhibited in her cardiovascular apparatus the effects of sustained attempts to compensate for her inadequacies made especially apparent to her by the achievements of her more fortunate sister.

ATTITUDES

Dealing further with the question, "Why is one organ and not another involved in a reaction pattern?" It may be suggested that the pattern of response depends in large part on the individual's conscious or unconscious perception of the situation. The latter would in turn depend on his point of view ingrained first by heredity, then by culture, and the sum total of his previous experiences. Attitudes in those with conspicuous manifestations of stress have been carefully studied by Grace and Graham (29,

30). The attitude may be conscious and verbally expressed or, more usually, unconscious, or at least unrecognized.

Although it is often difficult to elicit remarks that indicate attitudes because of a patient's inarticulateness or lack of vocabulary, when adequate expression is possible, it is striking how bodily reactions evoked during stress, are associated with highly specific verbalizations.

Exposure to the attitudes and behavior of parents may result in the development of predictable attitudes in their children. Also, many patients with the same stress manifestations are found to have had certain common experiences. Their reactions thus being conditioned by earlier exposure, similar situations encountered later evoke the learned response. Indeed, when the responses persist over years they may become an aspect of the "character" of the person. But even in the absence of infantile or childhood exposure, certain adult life experiences may possess intrinsically high potentiality for evoking particular bodily changes. Thus the development of new reaction patterns is always possible—a possibility that may be profitably exploited in therapy (see Chapter VI).

Grace and Graham (29) elicited the individual's attitude by having him make a statement at the time of the occurrence of a symptom of what he felt was happening to him, and what he wanted to do about it. Statements made *at the time* of the occurrence were important, since often an individual expressed himself quite another way about the precipitating event at a later date. Over-all words indicating the emotional component of their reaction such as "anger," "resentment," "sickness," etc. were required to be further defined and explained.

Urticaria occurred when certain individuals saw themselves as being mistreated. This mistreatment in any one of them might take the form of something said to him or something done to him. He was preoccupied entirely with what was happening to him, and was not thinking of retaliation or of any solution to his problem. As indicated earlier, typical statements were: "They did a lot of things to me and I couldn't do anything about it." "I was taking a beating." "My mother was hammering on me." "The boss cracked a whip over me." "My fiancee knocked me down and walked all over me, but what could I do?"

In most cases, the attitude was in some sense a description of the function of the physiological process with which it was associated. Thus, vasodilatation is the reaction of the skin to trauma. Wheals may appear when vasodilatation is intense. The patient with urticaria felt that he was receiving a blow, and that there was nothing he could do about it.

Eczema occurred when given individuals felt that they were being interfered with or prevented from doing something, and could think of no way to deal with the frustration. Preoccupation in a particular patient was with the interference and the persons or things thwarting him, rather than with the goals or aims. Typical statements were: "I want to make my mother understand, but I can't." "I couldn't do what I wanted but there wasn't anything I could do about it." "It upset me because it interfered with what I wanted to do." "I felt terribly frustrated."

In addition, however, minor urticarial reactions or exacerbations of eczema occurred when a particular individual felt that he was being looked at and had no response to make—the feeling commonly called "embarrassment." An additional feature in many instances was the aggression directed toward the self, expressed in the statement, "I take it out on myself."

Cold and moist hands occurred when particular individuals felt that they should undertake some kind of activity even though they might not know precisely what to do. Typical statements were: "I wanted to hit him." "I just had to do something." "Something ought to be done." "I wanted to do something." Raynaud's disease is the phenomenon of cold, moist hands carried to the extreme. The action contemplated by those with Raynaud's disease was characteristically a hostile one. Typical statements were: "I wanted to hit him." "I wanted to put a knife through him." "I wanted to strangle him."

Cold skin under these circumstances is the result of cutaneous vasoconstriction (31, 32). Its occurrence in an individual who is contemplating some kind of action possibly represents the functioning of a mechanism to raise body temperature by reducing heat loss. That an elevated body temperature is desirable for the active organism is suggested by the fact that the elevation occurs with a standard amount of exercise whether heat loss is experimentally facilitated or retarded (33).

Vasomotor rhinitis occurred when specific individuals were facing a situation with the wish that they didn't have to do anything about it, or that it would go away, or that somebody else would take over the responsibility. The essential feature was the desire to have nothing to do with the situation, to deal with it by excluding it. Typical statements were: "I wanted them to go away." "I didn't want to have anything to do with it." "I wanted to blot it all out; I wanted to build a wall between him and me." "I wanted to hole up for the winter." "I wanted to go to bed and pull the sheets up over my head," a statement that suggests a subconscious desire to suffocate himself?

The reaction of the respiratory mucous membrane to a noxious agent is to exclude it by swelling of the membrane with consequent narrowing of the passageway, and to dilute it and wash it out by hypersecretion (34). When these changes are limited to the nose, the reaction is called vasomotor rhinitis; when they are sufficiently widespread to include the bronchi, so that wheezing occurs, the name "asthma" is applied (35-37).

Asthma occurred in association with attitudes like those accompanying vasomotor rhinitis, but in asthma the feelings seemed more intense. While attacks of asthma were almost invariably accompanied by vasomotor rhinitis, the reverse was not true. In short, the two conditions seem to be essentially part of the same reaction, the difference being one of intensity.

Diarrhea was encountered in association with a wish to get on with and be done with, or to get rid of something or somebody connected with it. Typical statements were: "If the war was only over with." "I wanted to get done with it." "I wanted to get finished with it." "I've got too many responsibilities. I can't possibly do all that is expected of me."

Defecation is a way of ridding the body of substances which have been taken in but are no longer useful. Diarrhea, or frequent defecation, then, occurs in the setting of an intense desire to get something finished or to dispose of too heavy a load.

Constipation accompanied an attitude of grim determination to carry on, even though faced with an insoluble problem. Typical statements were: "I have to keep on with this, but I know I'm not going to like it." "It's a lousy job, but it's the best I can do." "This marriage is never going to be any better but I won't quit."

Constipation is a phenomenon of "holding on" without change. This corresponds to the patient's attitude of trying to continue with things as they are, without hope of immediate improvement (38, 39), and to the grimly uttered statement, "I have to hang on to what I've got."

Nausea and vomiting occurred when certain individuals were confronted by a fact which they wished had never happened. Such a patient, for example, was preoccupied with the mistake he had made, rather than with what he should have done instead. Usually, he felt responsible for what had happened. Typical statements were: "I wish it hadn't happened." "I was sorry I did it." "I wish things were the way they were before." "I made a mistake." "I shouldn't have listened to him."

Vomiting corresponds to the patient's efforts to restore things to their original situation as if nothing had ever happened.

Arterial hypertension occurred when individuals felt that they constantly must be prepared to meet all possible threats. Typical statements were: "I had to be ready for anything." "It was up to me to take care of all the worries." "Nobody is ever going to beat me, I'm ready for anything." "I've been sitting on the lid all my life, all ready for the explosion."

Low back pain was related to a desire to carry out some action involving movement of the entire body, but without the actual carrying out of such activity. The activity in question was usually walking or running away. Typical statements were: "I just wanted to walk out of the house." "I wanted to run away." "I wanted to get out of there." "I felt like taking a flying leap off that island." Other workers have been impressed that the sufferer with backache considers his "load too heavy,"—"they are expecting too much of me,"—"they have given me too much to do" (40).

The backache which accompanies the desire of the individual to "walk out" of his situation is possibly consequent on the tension of the lumbar muscles, fixing the spinal column in preparation for action (41). It has been shown that thinking about lifting a weight is associated with increased electrical activity in the appropriate muscle (42). It has also been demonstrated that sustained contraction of skeletal muscles can be painful (43).

In later studies, Graham et al. (30, 44, 45) confirmed most of their earlier inferences. Experiments were carried out in healthy volunteers under hypnosis to whom "pathogenic" attitudes of hives, Raynauds syndrome and hypertension were suggested. Measurements of skin temperature reflected a rise in association with the suggested hives attitude and a fall with the suggested Raynaud's syndrome attitude. When the hypertension attitude was suggested, the significant bodily change was a rise in diastolic blood pressure.

The focus on the recognition of attitudes grew out of earlier studies indicating that persons with certain stress manifestations such as migraine and other vascular headaches had a surprisingly large number of personality features in common which made it appear as though the bodily changes, personality features and reactions were linked (46). It was appreciated that there were individuals with these personality features who did not have the bodily changes or at least did not complain of them, and, on the other hand, that there were individuals who had the bodily complaint who did not possess all of the significant personality features. A later modification of this thesis with an attempt to bridge the difficulties encountered, emphasized a few conspicious attitudes of the patient, i.e., the expressed desire for non-participation of the patient with vasomotor rhinitis and asthma (34), and in the patient with migraine, dread of being found wrong, associated with striving to gain approval by working longer and harder than others.

There is no striking external similarity among the life situations which exacerbate a particular bodily response or disease episode; neither, inversely, is the same situation always associated with attacks. On the other hand, intensive observation of the patient's behavior, his manner of perceiving a situation and his attitudes oftentimes reveals them to be closely correlated to symptoms. Although there are semantic problems in evaluating a specificity hypothesis (47) further pursuit in this direction would appear to be profitable.

SUMMATIVE EFFECTS OF A VARIETY OF
STIMULUS SITUATIONS

As pointed out in Chapter III, the same protective reaction pattern may be elicited by a variety of stimuli. The ejection-riddance pattern of colonic hyperfunction for instance can be elicited by local irritants and bacteria as well as by symbolic threats to the individual's integrity or well-being. Not only do these various stimuli exert an additive effect, but one may prepare the soil for the other, thus increasing the individual's susceptibility. For example, there is evidence that the hyperemia and increased fragility of the colonic mucosa, occurring in association with suppressed anger and frustration may provide favorable circumstances for invasion by amoebae and other parasites (48 and 39). A kindred phenomenon was studied in detail on the nasal mucous membranes of pollen-sensitive individuals (49) as pointed out in Chapter III. It was found that the likelihood of an attack of hay fever after inhalation of standard quantities of pollen often depended upon whether or not there was pre-existing nasal hyperfunction in reaction to other stressful situations (Fig. 14, p. 58).

Moreover, in studies of the skin, pain and ischemia of the digits was found to depend not only upon the vasoconstriction resulting from low environmental temperatures, but also upon that accompanying anxiety and hostility (50, 51). Very dramatic indeed may be the additive phenomena resulting from effects of mechanical irritation of the skin and those associated with sustained resentment. Not only were hives induced by situational stimuli alone, but when such stimuli were inadequate to induce an observable change in the skin a wheal would result from slight mechanical stimulation, such as stroking or contact with tight clothing. A variety of non-specific agents may contribute to the outward show of dermatoses when the skin is already in such a state of increased sensitivity. Moreover the sensitivity of the skin to chemical agents changes so that amounts of histamine which under one set of emotionally meaningful circumstances produce no response whatever, may under others, evoke urticarial reactions. Indeed, during periods of stress, skin and mucous membranes may exhibit to a host of foods, pollens, drugs and similar chemical agents, an increased sensitivity not present during periods of relative tranquillity.

FRAGMENTATION OF PROTECTIVE PATTERNS: THE PRINCIPLE OF PARSIMONY

In adults, noxious symbols seldom evoke a full-blown integrated protective response. Instead, the reaction pattern is likely to be fragmented. Despite excessive and sustained local reactions, there is none the less a kind of parsimony in that the extreme response may be sharply limited in distribution. For example, defensive reactions involving the airways may include chiefly the nose and a few structures below the nasal airways, excluding the lung, diaphragm, the eyes and mouth. Or, on the other hand, in the asthmatic, the upper airways may be relatively little involved. Again, the esophagus involved in a pattern of rejection, as manifest in cardiospasm (52) may allow nothing to enter the stomach, whereas the gastrointestinal tract below that point may be functioning adequately. The terminal portion of the large bowel may be involved in an ejection pattern, while the ileum and the jejunum are functioning in an average way.

Hyperfunction of the stomach and duodenum may be associated with average function in adjacent portions of the gastrointestinal tract. During the hyperdynamic circulatory reaction to stress, heart rate, peripheral vasomotor function and stroke volume may augment together, or one or more may increase independently of the others. Again, hypodynamic circulatory responses may involve separately heart rate, peripheral vasomotor function and stroke volume.

In the respiratory system, a protective reaction of shutting out, washing away and neutralizing assaults or threats has been identified, involving the airways from the nose to the diaphragm and all the accessory muscles of breathing. The facial muscles, the tear ducts and even the eyes, become implicated as in weeping. The nasal airways become occluded and their mucous membranes become hyperemic and turgescent. Mucus is vigorously secreted as the bronchi become narrowed so that edematous and wet mucous membranes block the movement of gases. The diaphragm may be contracted, limiting ventilation: In combination with the diaphragmatic spasm, the esophagus may be occluded. This complete biological pattern of exclusion is seldom seen. Far more commonly only a part of the pattern is used, any of the phenomena mentioned occurring alone or in combination with some of the others.

These specific and highly localized responses indicate a parsimony in reaction to threats. Such parsimony is the keynote of an adaptive reaction in which the engendered feelings of security are out of proportion to the protection afforded by the response (53).

Parsimony is in keeping with the general principle that an individual will raise no more defenses than are necessary to attain a feeling of safety. It is noted that often when a bodily defense pattern is well established the subject may exhibit an extraordinary degree of tranquility (i.e., the seeming tranquility of the patient with serious ulcerative colitis). This may lead to the initially erroneous conclusion that the subject has no serious adaptive difficulties.

On the other hand, an extremely threatened individual may exhibit no significant bodily or emotional reactions other than, for example, hand washing and excessive bathing, as if cleanliness would protect him from everything. Even more devoid of bodily protective patterns is the individual who is dedicated to the proposition that he is a king or even a god, and thus rests in the security of unchallenged superiority. Investigation often reveals that the same individual may have used from time to time one or many protective bodily reaction patterns, eventually retreating into a more comfortable state of unreality. Also, such a person's unreal adaptive system may decompensate and a host of bodily reactions, fears and even terror become manifest to himself and others.

Despite complaints and troublesome symptoms, the adjustment represented by the protective reaction pattern is not without value to the individual. Though often clumsy, inappropriate, misdirected and sometimes containing mixtures of patterns, such protective reactions afford relative tranquillity and in many instances, a workable and useful life adjustment, becoming a

nuisance or menace only when they threaten the goal or survival
(18, 21).

THE SIGNIFICANCE OF THE EVENT AS A DETERMINANT
OF THE NATURE OF THE PROTECTIVE
REACTION PATTERN

Common experience presents numerous instances of persons with extremely troublesome symptom complexes, who, in
the face of a catastrophe or during great grief or exultation,
become remarkably free of symptoms, only to have them recur
when the crisis has passed. For example, a remarkable remission
of symptoms from a peptic ulcer was observed in a forty-year-old
physician during and for about a week after a harrowing experience. While sailing in a small boat he was caught in a storm,
and nearly lost his life as well as that of his companion. For two
years prior to the crisis created by the storm, he had suffered
symptoms of peptic ulcer, especially troublesome during the
stress of his daily responsibilities and anxieties.

Freedom from symptoms has also been observed under
extreme circumstances that evoked different and overriding reaction patterns. Thus Groen (54, 55) cared for and studied a
group of Amsterdam citizens during the period before World
War II, then followed them in concentration camp after the
invasion of Holland and finally cared for them again as civilians,
following the end of hostilities. This group included individuals
with peptic ulcer who, because they were Jews, were exposed to
indignities, deprivations and severe threats and hazards in concentration camps. The majority had been successful merchants,
or professional persons with active competitive careers. Most of
them lost the symptoms and manifestations of peptic ulcer during
their harrowing experiences in concentration camp when none
knew whether they would survive the day. They felt and exhibited
great fear and hatred. The latter was focused especially on fellow
Jewish prisoners of other nationalities: i.e., the Dutch "hated"
the Polish Jews, the Polish "hated" the French and the Dutch,
etc. There was much snarling, bickering, quarreling, snatching,
stealing, fighting and overt display of hostility toward their

guards. They ceased striving to maintain ethical standards, were in no sense "ambitious," expressed their feelings openly and freely and considered the acquisition of a little extra food or comfort a major triumph. On the other hand, they were for the most part emotionally supported by their spouses at this time. When these individuals were once more restored to the habits, customs and attitudes of civilian life, manifestations of peptic ulcer recurred in many.

One of the rare recurrences of ulcer with hemorrhage in the concentration camp was observed in an idealistic university professor who attempted to live up to the dignity of his role as a leader in society. On the other hand, diarrhea, which, as noted above, is associated with overwhelming situations, was common in the concentration camp even among those formerly constipated. But few patients with ulcerative colitis improved; indeed one of the latter became worse and died.

Groen (56) relates another striking instance of a specific response in terms of the significance of a stressful situation. During the German occupation of Holland, a young Dutch girl with diabetes was being courted by a young man who was not acceptable to her parents. On a number of occasions violent quarrels in the family, especially between the girl and her mother, grew out of this lack of approval. On these occasions, the patient developed ketosis and sometimes approached coma.

This young woman was employed as an office worker, and, on one dark afternoon, was obliged to switch on the electric light over her desk. The German military regulations imposed a severe penalty on any individual who made it possible for enemy planes over the city at night to see light. It was therefore her grave responsibility to turn off the light, but, since the day had grown brighter when she left the office, she forgot to do so. With nightfall the windows of the office became brilliantly illuminated. A friend, who had seen the police enter the office and knew that they were about to arrest her, hurried to the girl's home to give the alarm. She was truly terrified by the implications of her act and was almost in panic. Under these circumstances she developed no manifestations of ketosis or other augmentation of her metabolic disturbances, but did develop violent diarrhea.

The special meaning of a change in personality of one member of a tightly knit family to others in that unit was described by Koskoff (57). The adjustments made necessary by the return to their midst of a central family figure, whose behavior following lobotomy was seriously altered, precipitated a peptic ulcer in one member.

A group of missionaries in the Far East with migraine headache completely lost their migraine attacks when incarcerated in Japanese concentration camps, when they were freed of the need to maintain standards or achieve goals, even though they suffered many deprivations and even experienced torture. Protective reaction patterns are perhaps less likely to be evoked in prison camps, and in wartime and combat situations where there is an unusual opportunity for the free expression of hatred and hostility. Furthermore, such reaction patterns are most likely to occur in situations directly connected with or symbolic of the individual's own goals, his mode of attaining them and the conflicts thus created.

Therefore, the nature of the protective reaction pattern is determined by the significance of the situation to the implicated individual. A vivid example was provided in a surprising way during an investigation of subjects with cold hands and Raynaud's syndrome. The subjects were required to read a ghoulish account of automobile accidents entitled "And Sudden Death" by J. C. Furnas. Most subjects developed cold hands when they read the article. One subject, an attractive seventeen-year-old girl, responded to the story with only modest fall in her finger temperature (Fig. 43). Accordingly, she was asked to read what was considered to be a neutral piece of literature, President Franklin D. Roosevelt's speech dedicating the Jersey City Medical Center (51). As she read this address her hands became icy cold. The puzzled investigators ascertained that this girl had been at an impressionable age of eleven when Roosevelt was elected President. Her father and brothers had been out of work and there had been no meat on the table. After the election, her father and brothers found work and the family fortunes suddenly improved. In her childish mind (and unaware of the pitfalls of experimental design) she attributed this coincidence to the fact that Mr.

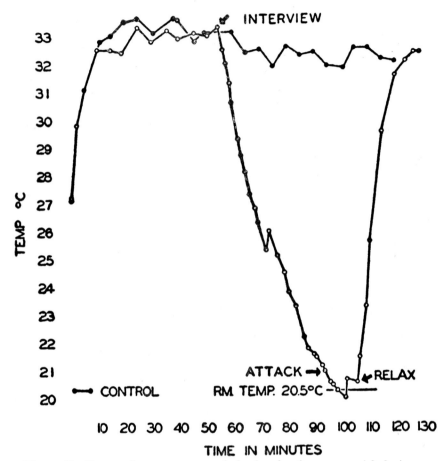

Figure 43. Changes in temperature of the hands of a young girl during a stressful interview.

Roosevelt was in the White House. However—and this illustrates the perversity of human nature—her father and brothers campaigned vigorously at the next election in favor of the Republicans. When at dinner they said uncomplimentary things about Mr. Roosevelt, the girl felt such a conflict of loyalties between her father and her beloved president that she often left the table without eating.

In the experimental situation, she had read "And Sudden Death" without turning a hair (or you might say, without cooling her hands) because she was used to reading the *New York*

Daily News. The dedication of the Jersey City Medical Center had no intrinsic emotional meaning, but it symbolized the continuing conflict of loyalties so important to her.

Rhythms and Cycles

Dramatic aspects of living matter relevant to the organization of reaction patterns are the long and short rhythms and cycles of biological activity and responsivity (58, 59). They often correspond to cosmic events and thereby come around yearly, monthly, or daily. The periods of other cycles are shorter still. In a study of the excretion of salt and water in healthy men, Mock and associates observed that the equilibrium of intake and output oscillated in fairly broad waves with retention for a few days followed by diuresis (60) (Fig. 44). When a potent diuretic was given to an individual at the end of the diuretic limb of his cycle, it had far less effect than when administered

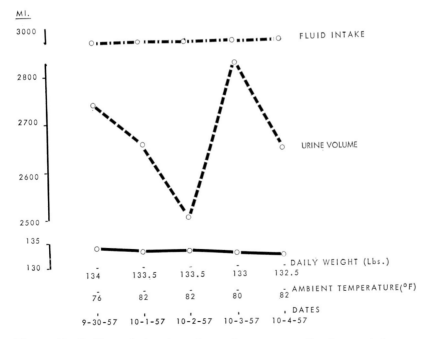

Figure 44. Cyclic variation in urine volume over a five-day period on a constant water and salt intake.

after a period of retention. Similarly, gastric motor activity was found to describe a cycle in the unfed human, coming on about every three hours and lasting twenty minutes. We found that a cholinergic drug was relatively ineffective in setting up contractions if given shortly after the end of a spontaneously occurring cycle of activity (61). Thus, man's responsiveness to drugs is greater at some times than at others. It may also be that our tendency to be sick is greater at some times than others. Halberg, for example, found that the capacity of a mouse to withstand an endotoxin produced by Escherichia coli varies with the circadian cycle of light and darkness. A dose that killed 85 per cent of mice at their "subjective noon" killed less than 5 per cent at their "subjective midnight" (62).

Pavlov observed that conditioned responses in dogs may exhibit cyclic variation in magnitude of response to standard stimuli (63).

Richter has extensively studied cyclical behavior in rats such as eating and running (64). The variations within the cycle were found to be great, for example running activity varied from next to nothing to fifteen miles per day. A striking feature of Richter's studies was that the cycles were very little subject to modification by circumstances or any kind of change in receptor activity. Thus, the animals were blinded and deafened without modifying the cycles. Their control also appeared to be independent of the endocrine glands. Removal of pituitary, thyroid and adrenals failed to modify the cycles to any significant extent. Only surgical division of the two hemispheres was found capable of disrupting the fixed cyclical patterns. For man, it is important that his vulnerability varies with the phases of his inherent cycles. This is made dramatically evident in the case of the long airplane flight which involves a time change of several hours. Shortly after such a flight, not only is the rhythm of sleep and wakefulness disrupted, but one's ability to cope and one's sensitivity to a variety of "assaults" may be greatly altered. The long flight illustrates another feature of man—namely that at least some of his cycles may be modified so that he becomes after a few days habituated to a new time cycle. Returning suddenly to the old one will reproduce the disruption.

The circadian cycle of adrenal function in man is more difficult to modify and may have importance with respect to vulnerability to environmental forces. A very familiar cycle associated with changing vulnerability and susceptibility to symptoms and bodily disorders is the menstrual cycle. The failure to adjust to menstruation by maintaining high levels of work performance may be, in those subject to vascular headache, the setting of attacks during this period. Even psychotic behavior in man has been observed to recur according to a predictable cycle (65). In short, the capacity of the individual to adapt is not a static function, but a varying one expressed as fluctuation in energy, drive and courage.

MENTAL MECHANISMS AND DISTURBANCES IN BRAIN FUNCTION AS ASPECTS OF ADAPTATION

Among the mental processes involved in organized adaptive reactions is depression with excessive grief or disguised hostility; the severe distorting reactions exemplified by the schizophrenic disorders in which a withdrawn individual's image of the environment may become radically altered; the panic reactions; the phobias; the amnesias coupled with loss of motility and sensory functions; and the obsessive compulsive "perfectionistic" and "ruminative" reactions. There is commonly much admixture.

Inter-related mechanisms include repression, a process whereby the individual adapts, by eliminating from awareness, a body of experience that is painful or dangerous. This is linked with forgetting or losing from awareness to the extent that the incident cannot be recalled by ordinary means. Also included is the process of rejection or the adaptation to danger by denying its existence or if recognizing it, at the same time assuming for oneself a position of detachment and aloofness. Allied to this is a withdrawal or god-like superiority as mentioned above so that human and personal travail is looked at from afar.

Such processes substitute in a sense for more direct or apparently appropriate reactions perhaps because the individual finds himself unable to face the reality and deal with it. Thus, they recall the part reactions discussed in an earlier section resembling the proverbial behavior of the ostrich who when in danger hides his head but leaves the rest of his body exposed.

An analogous process of organizing an adaptation is one of substituting an acceptable though crippling fantasy, often of a sensory or motor disability, for an unacceptable and painful fact. This is exemplified by the soldier who develops a reversible palsy in the arm when called upon to enter battle. Also illustrative is the development of "pain" in a woman, which eliminates the possibility of sexual intercourse with an unacceptable partner. Akin to this mechanism is "over-reaction" to a minor pain or unusual sensation as a dangerous implication which cannot be directly met. Thus, a woman, after having had a brain tumor removed continued to overcomplain about minor disturbances in function of the eyes while she became increasingly disabled with myelogenous leukemia and diabetes. Until the day of her death, she focused her numerous complaints on the "brain tumor" and the possibility of its recurrence, but never mentioned her cachexia, anemia, weakness and bleeding gums.

These mental mechanisms alone or in combination may be linked with appropriate bodily adaptation patterns or may occur independently in the category of ideation and fantasy. Though the neuraxis is involved in the integration of all patterns of adaptation, the functions of the brain as an organ may not be altered by the process. However, there are adaptive reaction patterns which disorganize brain functions and become manifest as serious disturbances in consciousness. This was demonstrated in conditioning experiments in humans (66, 67). Repeated exposure of the subjects to bright light produced a predictable change, i.e., alpha blocking, in the E.E.G. Auditory stimuli failed to do so. When the auditory stimulus was presented repeatedly before the visual stimulus, however, the sound temporarily but predictably acquired the property of the light to suppress alpha activity (Fig. 45). In subjects with structural brain damage, the linkage between sound and light occurred much less frequently. A similar failure of the conditioning process was observed in intact subjects during severe anxiety and prolonged periods of difficulty in life adjustment. These studies imply that failure of the brain to respond in the usual fashion to external stimuli

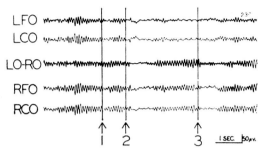

Figure 45. (a) Electroencephalogram of normal subject before appearance of temporary cerebral connections. Arrow 1 indicates appearance of sound; arrow 2, appearance of light; and arrow 3, disappearance of alpha activity following appearance of light.

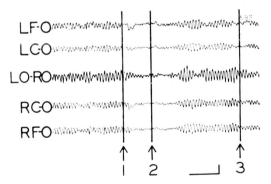

Figure 45. (b) Electroencephalogram of normal subject demonstrating presence of temporary cerebral connection. In this example, sound (arrow 1) is followed by disappearance of alpha activity before the appearance of the light (arrow 2).

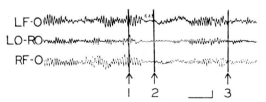

Figure 45. (c) Electroencephalogram of another normal subject demonstrating presence of a temporary cerebral connection, as shown by disappearance of alpha activity following onset of sound (arrow 1) before the appearance of light (arrow 2).

may constitute a part of the inappropriate patterns of reaction to stressful circumstances. As discussed in Chapter III, it was even possible experimentally to evoke seizures in suitably susceptible subjects by a stress interview. (See Figs. 46 and 47.)

Other examples of electroencephalographic changes occurring as part of an adaptive reaction are provided by studies of those with narcolepsy, a syndrome featured by uncontrollable sleepiness, "sleep paralysis," episodes of extreme weakness during laughter and exceedingly vivid dreams containing incidents hard to distinguish from happenings occurring in the waking state (68). Such patients often give evidence of great conflict between needs for self-differentiation and acceptance of a binding pattern of life laid down by others. When topics of grave personal significance were introduced in an interview, the subjects studied by Barker (69, 70) and referred to earlier in Chap. III, showed changes in the brain waves in the direction of synchronization similar to those which occur during sleep, and concurrently exhibited the behavioral features of narcolepsy. The adaptation in this instance resulting in sleep may be said to alter brain function with the implied purpose of protecting the individual from the untoward effects of active participation.

Figuratively, there are in the neuraxis of vertebrates, two nervous systems, one within the other. The first is involved directly in the responses to afferent impulses from external stimuli. The second maintains the first in a proper state of excitation so that it can execute responses appropriately. The major neural structure involved is the internuncial neuron operating at all levels within the neuraxis with an important locus of activity in the midbrain (71, 72).

In this connection (73), it has been shown from the analysis of surface hyperalgesia that afferent impulses from noxious stimulation of the skin insufficiently strong to evoke pain, may, none the less, through the operation of the internuncial neurons, so augment excitation in the neuraxis as to cause subsequent painful stimuli to be felt as more intense (Fig. 48). Further, in patients with lesions giving rise to low-intensity sustained pain, threatening life experiences can so increase the general level of excitation that the pain is intensified and other adaptive reactions

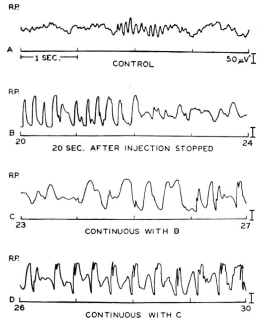

RP.

A ⊢—1 SEC.—⊣   CONTROL   50μV I

RP.

B 20   20 SEC. AFTER INJECTION STOPPED   24 I

RP.

C 23   CONTINUOUS WITH B   27 I

RP.

D 26   CONTINUOUS WITH C   30 I

Figure 46. EEG wave patterns during development of a major convulsion during sodium amytal interview. Monopolar recording through the 6-channel Grass machine. All illustrations from the right parietal lead with the usual amplification and filtering constant throughout. A, Control record before amytal was given. B, As the reaction passed from rage into the tonic phase of the convulsion. C, Overlapping continuation of B, showing the transition to D, end of the tonic phase with wave pattern similar to that described by Gibbs as "grand mal with petit mal component seizure."

are evoked. Since the reactions to painful noxious stimulation are so similar to those of other threatening situations, it is suggested that in a comparable way, the general excitatory state may be augmented by sustained threats. This would cause a heightened response to a host of relatively minor stressful situations.

The disturbance in brain function coupled with blurring of consciousness and, as well, unconsciousness in certain individuals with epilepsy were studied by Barker (70). Normal integrative activity represents one form of neuronal hyperactivity. The neurons, though hyperactive, are interrelated in such a fashion that potential discharges from a given area are asynchronous. On the other hand, the abnormal waves found in epileptics represent

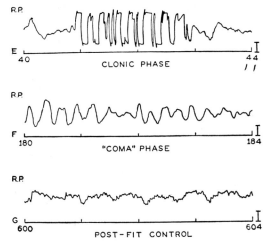

Figure 47. EEG during the further development of the convulsion shown in Figure 46. E, A clonic burst 41 seconds after the convulsion began. The high voltage threw the writing pens into the stops, producing the squared waves. F, Postconvulsive coma three minutes after the fit began. G, Ten minutes after the fit began and six minutes after recovery of consciousness. The absence of fast activity usually associated with the intravenous administration of sodium amytal is interesting.

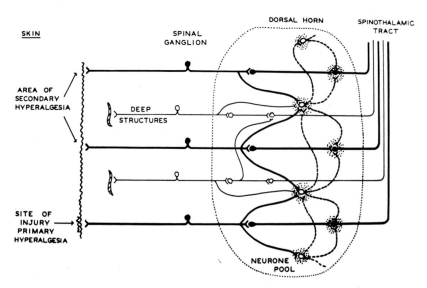

Figure 48. Schematic diagram suggesting the mechanism of secondary hyper-algesia. Central spread of excitation via internuncial neurons in the dorsal horn to involve connections from neighboring deep and superficial structures.

another form of neuronal hyperactivity. The neurons in this case are interrelated so that potential discharges are excessively synchronized. Barker showed that integrative activity in those with epilepsy is brought to a standstill (lapse of consciousness with excessive synchronization) by sudden conflicting and intensely distressing thoughts and feelings.

It is suggested that the neural equipment of some patients with epilepsy is such that the profound repression of rage is capable of disrupting cerebral function and interrupting mentation. At least in these instances, the adaptive processes involving repression are related to significant alterations in brain activity.

Structural Changes in the Brain as a Result of Adaptation

There is much to indicate that the brain itself, in integrating highest level adaptive responses, may be damaged as a consequence of improper interaction between organism and environment (74).

In men, and in some laboratory animals, the development of brain function may be retarded when in infancy they are deprived of suitable challenge, adequate stimulation, the protection of a parent, and opportunities for successful interaction with the environment. Infants and children have failed to mature when they have been raised in relentlessly hostile environments or in those permitting of no continuing human relationship (75). Although many aged persons continue to meet challenges adequately and maintain an active relationship with the world around them, it has often been pointed out that those who retire and withdraw themselves from challenging situations, often deteriorate rapidly when they are thus deprived of their work and social responsibilities.

In man, total isolation and severely restricted sensory stimulation are followed by temporary impairment of high level brain functions. Men subjected to the prolonged abuse and hatred of their fellows, as in prison, behave as though their heretofore actively functioning brains were severely damaged. They pass through predictable states of progressive impairment, comparable to the impairment observed in subjects with progressive loss of brain substance. Even when sleep and food are adequate, complete isolation, lack of opportunity to talk, repeated failure, frustration, and reviling by other men can cloud the mind and may make a man confabulate, become more suggestible, and cause him to rationalize behavior previously unacceptable (76).

The quantitative methods developed through the study of individuals with cerebral ablations permitted assessment of highest level brain function in ostensibly intact individuals who had experienced prolonged periods of unresolved difficulties in adaptation (77, 78). It was found that persons with no evidence of gross anatomic disease of the brain but who, for long periods had achieved no effective adaptation and had experienced longstanding anxiety and other disturbances in behavior and mood (both with and without bodily disorders), exhibited severe thinking and adaptive difficulties. Indeed, they performed in their usual lives and laboratory test procedures as though moderate and sometimes massive amounts of brain had been damaged or removed. Those with effective defenses such as blaming, rationalizing, sublimation, denying, pretending, or withdrawing from participation, showed less deterioration in brain function. But, when these defenses were no longer adequate or stress had been too prolonged, these individuals too, demonstrated a persisting impairment of highest level brain functions.

The observed "mass action" relationship between the highest level functions and the aggregates of neurons in the cerebral hemispheres may give a clue to the nature of the process. For highest level functions, the number and degree of orderly arrangement of nerve cells is of central importance, and the pattern of specific localized connections, so important for lower level functions, is of lesser significance. As pointed out earlier, order itself becomes the relevant attribute for understanding of the relationship between the neuron and the highest level functions.

BIBLIOGRAPHY

1. SANTAYANA, G.: *The Life of Reason; or, The Phases of Human Progress:* One-volume edition revised by the author in collaboration with Daniel Cory. New York, Scribner, 1954.
2. STRAUSS, M. G.: The climate for the cultivation of clinical rerearch. *New Eng. J. Med., 262*:805-810, 1960.

3. WHITEHEAD, A. N.: *Science and the Modern World* (Lowell Lectures). New York, MacMillan, 1925.
4. WOODGER, J. H.: *Biological Principles. A Critical Study.* New York, Harcourt, 1929.
5. EDDINGTON, A. S.: *The Nature of the Physical World* (Gifford Lectures, 1927).
6. KREBS, H. A.: *Excursion into Borderland of Biochemistry and Philosophy* (Herter Lecture). *Bull. Hopkins Hosp.*, 1954.
7. HALDANE, J. B. S., and PRIESTLEY, J. G.: *Respiration*, London, Oxford, 1935.
8. CANNON, W. B.: *The Wisdom of the Body.* New York, Norton, 1932.
9. SINNOTT, E. W.: *Matter, Mind and Man: The Biology of Human Nature.* New York, Harper, 1957.
10. BARNETT, S. A., EATON, J. D., and McCALLUM, H. M.: Physiological effects of "social stress" in wild rats—I. *J. Psychosom. Res.,* 3:1-11, 1958.
11. BARNETT, S. A., EATON, J. D., and McCALLUM, H. M.: Physiological effects of "social stress" in Wild Rats—II. *J. Psychosom. Res.,* 4:251-260, 1960.
12. BARNETT, S. A.: "Displacement" behavior and "psychosomatic" disorder. *Lancet,* 269:1203-1208, 1955.
13. TINBERGEN, N.: "Derived" activities: their causation, biological significance and emancipation during evolution. *Quart. Rev. Biol.,* 27:1-32, 1952.
14. COHEN, E. A.: *Human Behavior in the Concentration Camp.* London, Jonathan Cape, 1954.
15. WOLFF, H. G.: Protective reaction patterns and disease (Loeb Lecture) *Ann. Intern. Med.,* 27:944-969, 1947.
16. WOLFF, H. G.: Changes in vulnerability of tissue: An aspect of man's response to threat. The National Institute of Health, Annual Lectures, 1953, pp. 38-72. U.S. Dept. of Health, Education and Welfare. Publication #388.
17. HINKLE, L. E., and WOLFF, H. G.: The nature of man's adaptation to his total environment and the relation of this to illness. *Arch. Intern. Med. (Chicago),* 99:442-460, 1957.
18. WOLFF, H. G.: What hope does for man. Science and Humanity Section, *Saturday Rev.,* pp. 42-45, 1956 (Also reprinted and distributed by N. Y. State Committee on TB and P.H. and N. Y. State Heart Assoc., Inc.). Also see: Has Disease Meaning? *Soc. N. Y. Hosp. Rec.,* May 8, 1956, pp. 10-17.

19. WOLF, S.: A new view of disease. *Trans. Amer. Clin. Climat. Ass.*, *74*:168-175, 1963, *J.A.M.A.*, *184(2)*:129, 1963.

20. WOLF, STEWART: Life stress and patterns of disease. In: *The Psychological Basis of Medical Practice*, Harold Lief, Victor Lief, and Nina Lief, Eds. New York, Hoeber, 1963, Chap. 9, p. 109.

21. WOLF, S.: Disease as a way of life. Neural integration in systemic pathology. *Perspect. Biol. Med.*, pp. 288-305, Spring, 1961.

22. RICHTER, CURT: Domestication of the Norway rat and its implications for the problem of stress. *Proc. Ass. Res. Nerv. Ment. Dis.*, *29*:19, 1950.

23. RICHTER, CURT: The role played by the thyroid gland in the production of gross body activity. *Endocrinology*, *17*:73, 1933.

24. RICHTER, CURT: The effect of early gonadectomy on the gross body activity of rats. *Endocrinology*, *17*:445, 1933.

25. RICHTER, CURT: Cyclical phenomena produced in rats by section of the pituitary stalk and their possible relation to pseudo pregnancy. *Amer. J. Physiol.*, *106*:80, 1933.

26. SELYE, H., and FORTIER, C.: Adaptive reactions to stress. *Proc. Ass. Res. Nerv. Ment. Dis.*, *29*:3, 1950.

27. FLYNN, J. T., KENNEDY, M. A. K., and WOLF, S.: Essential hypertension in one of identical twins. An experimental study of cardiovascular reactions in the Y twins. *Proc. Ass. Res. Nerv. Ment. Dis.*, *29*:954, 1950.

28. SHELDON, S. H., and BALL, R.: Physical characteristics of the Y twins and their relation to hypertension. *Proc. Ass. Res. Nerv. Ment. Dis.*, *29*:962, 1950.

29. GRACE, W. J., and GRAHAM, D. T.: The specificity of the relation between attitudes and disease. *Psychosom. Med.*, *14*:243, 1952.

30. GRAHAM, D. T., LUNDY, R. M., BENJAMIN, L. S., KABLER, J. D., LEWIS, W. C., KUNISH, N. O., and GRAHAM, F. K.: Specific attitudes in initial interviews with patients having different "psychosomatic" disease. *Psychosom. Med.*, *24*:257, 1962.

31. BROBECK, JOHN R.: Regulation of energy exchange. In: *A Textbook of Physiology*. John Fulton, Ed. Philadelphia, Saunders, 1949.

32. HARDY, J. D.: Physiology of temperature regulation. *Physiol. Rev.*, *41*:521-606, 1961.

33. NIELSEN, M.: Die regulation der Korperterperatur bei Muskelarbeit. *Skand. Arch. Physiol.*, *79*:193, 1938.

34. HOLMES, T. H., GOODELL, H., WOLF, S., and WOLFF, H. G.: *The Nose: An Experimental Study of Reactions within the Nose in Human Subjects.* Springfield, Thomas, 1950.

35. FAULKNER, W. B.: X-ray evidence of emotional influence upon esophageal function. *Amer. J. Psychiat., 98*:227, 1941.

36. FAULKNER, W. B.: Effect of emotions upon diaphragmatic function; observations on five patients. *Psychosom. Med., 3*:187, 1941.

37. FAULKNER, W. B.: Influence of suggestion on size of bronchial lumen: Bronchoscopic study and report of one case. *Northwest Med., 40*:367, 1941.

38. ALMY, T. P., KERN, F., JR., and ABBOT, F. K.: Constipation and diarrhea as reactions to life stress. *Proc. Ass. Res. Nerv. Ment. Dis., 29*:724, 1950.

39. GRACE, W. J., WOLF, S., and WOLFF, H. G.: *The Human Colon. An Experimental Study Based on Direct Observation of Four Fistulous Subjects.* New York, Hoeber, 1951.

40. HOLMES, T. H., and WOLFF, H. G.: Life situations, emotions and backache. *Psychosom. Med., 14*:18-33, 1952.

41. STENDLER, A.: *Mechanics of normal and pathological locomotion in man.* Springfield, Thomas, 1935.

42. JACOBSON, E.: Electrophysiology of mental activities. *Amer. J. Physiol., 44*:677, 1932.

43. SIMONS, D. J., DAY, E., GOODELL, H., and WOLFF, H. G.: Experimental studies on headache: Muscles of the scalp and neck as sources of pain. *Proc. Ass. Res. Nerv. Ment. Dis., 23*:228, 1943.

44. GRAHAM, D. T., STERN, J. A., and WINKOUR, G.: Experimental investigation of the specificity of attitude hypothesis in psychosomatic disease. *Psychosom. Med., 20*:446, 1958.

45. GRAHAM, D. T., KABLER, J. D., and GRAHAM, F. K.: Physiological response to the suggestion of attitudes specific for hives and hypertension. *Psychosom. Med., 24*:159, 1962.

46. WOLFF, H. G.: *Headache and Other Head Pain.* New York, Oxford, 1948 and 1963.

47. KOGAN, W. S., DORPAT, T. L., and HOLMES, T. H.: Sematic problems in evaluating a specificity hypothesis in psychophysiologic relations. *Psychosom. Med., 27*:1, 1965.

48. GRACE, W. J., WOLF, S., and WOLFF, H. G.: Life situations, emotions and chronic ulcerative colitis. *J.A.M., 142*:1044, 1950.

49. HOLMES, T. H., TREUTING, T., and WOLFF, H. G.: Life situations, emotions and nasal disease: Evidence on summative effects exhibited in patients with hay fever. *Proc. Ass. Res. Nerv. Ment. Dis.*, 29:545, 1950. Also: *Psychosom. Med.*, 13:71, 1951.

50. GRAHAM, DAVID T.: The pathogenesis of hives: Experimental study of life situations, emotions and cutaneous vascular reactions. *Proc. Ass. Res. Nerv. Ment. Dis.*, 29:987, 1950.

51. MITTLEMAN, B., and WOLFF, H. G.: Affective states and skin temperature: Experimental study of subjects with "cold hands" and Raynaud's syndrome. *Psychosom. Med.*, 1:271-292, 1939.

52. WOLF, S., and ALMY, T. P.: Experimental observations on cardiospasm in man. *Gastroenterology*, 13:401, 1949.

53. WOLFF, H. G.: The mind-body relationship. In: *An Outline of Man's Knowledge*. New York, Doubleday, 1960, Chap. 2, pp. 43-72.

54. GROEN, J. J.: Personal Communication.

55. GROEN, J. J.: *Psychopathogenese van Ulcus Ventirculi et Duodeni*. Amsterdam, Scheltema and Holkema, 1947.

56. GROEN, J. J.: Personal communication.

57. KOSKOFF, Y. D., and WENIGER, F. L.: The adverse effect upon a family resulting from a radical change of personality in one member after frontal lobotomy. *Proc. Ass. Res. Nerv. Ment. Dis.*, 29:148, 1950.

58. PITTENDRIGH, COLIN S.: On temporal organization in living systems. *Harvey Lect., Serie, 56*:93, 1960-61.

59. RICHTER, CURT P.: Cyclic manifestations in the sleep curves of psychotic patients. *Arch. Nerul. Psychiat., 31*:149, 1934.

60. MOCK, D. C., JR., KYRIAKOPOULOS, A. A., CLARK, M. L., HAGANS, J. A., BRANDT, E. N., and WOLF, S.: Variability of diuretic response as influenced by the state of the organism. A note on the law of initial values. *Amer. J. Med. Sci., 238*:193-201, 1959.

61. WOLF, S.: *The Stomach*. New York, Oxford Univ. Press, 1965

62. HALBERG, F.: Temporal coordination of physiologic function. *Cold Spring Harbor Symposia on Quantitative Biology*, 25:289, 1960.

63. PAVLOV, I.: *Lectures on Conditioned Reflexes* trans. by W. H. Gantt. New York, Internat. Pub., 1928.

64. RICHTER, CURT P., JONES, G. S., and BISWANGER, L.: Periodic phenomena and the thyroid. I. Abnormal but regular cycles in behavior and metabolism produced in rats by partial radiothyroidectomy. *Arch. Neurol. Psychiat.,* *81(2)*:233-255, 1959.

65. RICE, KATHERINE, R.: Regular forty to fifty day cycle of psychotic behavior in a 14 year old boy. *Arch. Neurol. Psychiat., 51*:478, 1944.

66. WELLS, C. E., and WOLFF, H. G.: Formation of temporary cerebral connections in normal and brain damaged subjects. *Neurology, 10*:335-340, 1960.

67. WELLS, C. E., and WOLFF, H. G.: Electrographic evidence of impaired brain function in chronically anxious patients. *Science, 131*:1671-1672, 1960.

68. BARKER, WAYNE, and WOLF, S.: Experimental induction of grand mal seizure during the hypnoidal state induced by sodium amytal. *Amer. J. Med. Sci., 214*:600, 1947.

69. BARKER, W., and BARKER, S.: Experimental production of human convulsive brain potentials by stress induced effects upon neural integrative function: Dynamics of the convulsive reaction to stress. *Proc. Ass. Res. Nerv. Ment. Dis., 29*:90, 1950.

70. BARKER, WAYNE: Studies in epilepsy: Personality pattern, situational stress and the symptoms of narcolepsy. *Psychosom. Med., 10*:193, 1948.

71. MAGOUN, H. W.: An activating system in the brain stem. *Harvey Lect., 46,* 1951-52.

72. LORENTE DE NO, RAFAEL: Personal communications and Analysis of the activity of the chains of internuncial neurons. *J. Neurophysiol., 1*:207, 1938.

73. HARDY, J. D., WOLFF, H. G., and GOODELL, H.: Experimental evidence on the nature of cutaneous hyperalgesia. *J. Clin. Invest., 29*:115, 1950.

74. CHAPMAN, L., HINKLE, L. E., JR., and WOLFF, H. G.: Human ecology, disease and schizophrenia. *Amer. J. Psychiat., 117*: 193-204, 1960.

75. GOLDFARB, WILLIAM: Emotional and intellectual consequences of psychologic deprivation in infancy: A re-evaluation. In: *Psychopathology of Childhood.* New York, Grune and Stratton, 1955.

76. HINKLE, L. E., and WOLFF, H. G.: Communist interrogation and indoctrination of "Enemies of the State." Analysis of methods used by the Communist state police (a special report). *Arch. Neurol. Psychiat.*, *76*:115-174, 1956.

77. CHAPMAN, L., and WOLFF, H. G.: The cerebral hemispheres and the highest integrative functions of man. *Arch. Neurol.*, *1*:357-424, 1959.

78. CHAPMAN, L., THETFORD, W. N., BERLIN, L., GUTHRIE, T., and WOLFF, H. G.: Highest integrative functions in man during stress, Chap. XXI. In: *The Brain and Human Behavior*, Baltimore, Williams & Wilkins, 1958. *Proc. Ass. Res. Nerv. Ment. Dis.*, *36*:491-534, 1958.

Chapter V

THE BRAIN AND THE ADAPTIVE PROCESS

Evolution of Man's Knowledge of the Functions of the Brain (1-5)

Ancient Hindus and Chinese conceived of human attributes having to do with the spirit, with personality, feeling, sensation and mind, as being seated mainly in the organs of the chest or abdomen, and more on one side of the body than the other. Considered to be vaporous, these attributes were said to enter the body mainly through the mouth and airways and with death to leave from the top of the skull, through that portion last to ossify in infancy.

While prevailing Greek and early Christian concepts embraced such assumptions, Aristotle (384-322 B.C.) pronounced the heart to be the seat of the spirit, and his opinion influenced Western thought well into the European Renaissance. There was a series of shifts of the "seat of the soul" within the chest and abdomen, but mainly the heart was the preferred organ. The blood itself was also suggested. A less dominant Greek view placed the seat of the soul in the head.

Aristotle attached no importance to the brain but all to the blood vessels and the heart. This noble organ was for him the site of those powers which constitute the vital principle of the soul. It was the center of the processes of nutrition, sensation, thought, movement, and heat production in the body. Whereas Plato and others before him allocated these functions to different organs, particularly the heart, brain, and liver, Aristotle concentrated them all in the heart—the "acropolis of the body," as he called it. Of the brain, Aristotle wrote:

> "The vital spirit is distributed in the body throughout the blood vessels to all the organs of the body, vitalizing them. The one great exception to this is the brain, which is bloodless and

therefore insensitive and cold . . . The sensations of the animal, in particular man, depend upon the balance of the intensity of heat arising from the heart and the cooling process of the brain. Animals lower or less noble than man have insufficient brain to effect optimal cooling. Man's superior intelligence depends on the fact that his large brain is capable of keeping the heart cool enough for optimal mental activity" (6).

The degree to which even some of the Greeks found Aristotle's views unattractive is indicated by the comments of Galen (A. D. 130-201). When referring to Aristotle, he said, "I blush even today to quote his opinion." Galen rescued the work of several Alexandrians who had shown that the brain was part of the nervous system. He suggested, furthermore, that the brain was the locus of sensation and thought and that the "psychic pneuma," or animal spirits, were created in a knot of blood vessels at the base of the organ. He postulated that the watery fluid contained in the sizable chambers between parts of the brain transmitted these spirits to the spinal cord and thence via the nerves to the body generally. A valvelike arrangement between the chambers of the brain supposedly regulated the ebb and flow of the fluid and so influenced sensation and movement.

According to Galen, the "natural spirits," the products of nutrition, passed from the liver and the gut to the heart and were there modified by the material from the lungs. A portion of the resultant product, known as the "vital spirits," was passed to the head. Here, within the rich collection of blood vessels at the base of the brain, a watery distillate was recovered and mixed with air that supposedly entered the cranial cavity through the porous base of the skull above the nose. This "psychic pneuma" was then collected and circulated in the chambers of the brain. The by-products of the process were said to be drained off via the stalk of the pituitary into the nasal cavity.

By the fourth century A. D., this ingenious Galenic conception of the circulation of "psychic pneuma" within the chambers of the brain had been much modified. Saint Augustine (A. D. 354-430), among others, held that the three ventricles of the brain each individually contained "psychic pneuma" with special qualities. Indeed, some of the Aristotelian faculties were identified with the watery contents of the respective chambers, but not with the substance of the brain. Thus, in the anterior chamber close to a common sensory accumulation from the sense organs of the head and body were fantasy and imagination; in the middle chamber were reason, judgment, cogitation, estimation and thought, and in the posterior chamber were memory and motion, but movement of the fluid from chamber to chamber was the basis of much of behavior and thought. Passion and emotions were not included. This view persisted as the dominant one for a thousand years. Even William Harvey (1578-1657), who so elegantly demonstrated the nature of the heart's action and the circulation of the blood and who detected that reflexes involving the nervous system were implicated in sensation and motion, held to the Aristotelian view that the apparatus of feeling is in the heart and blood.

Descartes (1596-1650) did, however, link the substance of the brain with its function; but to the pineal body, a small insignificant protrusion within the chambers of the brain bathed by the contained fluids of the ventricles, he attributed the function of being the chief regulating organ of the soul. The following quotation exemplifies Descartes' position:

"The soul is really joined to the whole body, and we cannot properly speaking, say that it is in any one of its parts to the exclusion of the others—the body being unitary, i.e., in some fashion indivisible, in virtue of the disposition of its organs which are so related each to the others, that when any one of them is removed, the whole body is rendered defective. Again, the soul is of such a nature that it has no relation to extension, nor to the dimensions or to other properties of the matter composing the body, but only to the whole assemblage of its organs, as appears from our inability to think of the half or the third of a soul, or of its occupying a space. It does not become smaller on the removal of a part of the body. When, however, the assemblage of the bodily organs disintegrates, it itself, in its entirety, withdraws from the body . . .

"There is a small gland in the brain in which the soul exercises its function more specifically than in its other parts. We have also to bear in mind that although the soul is joined to the whole body, there is yet in the body a certain part in which it exercises its function more specifically than in all the others. It is a matter of common belief that this part is the brain, or probably the heart—the brain because of its relation to the senses, the heart because it is there we feel the passions. But on carefully examining the matter I seem to find evidence that the part of the body in which the soul exercises its functions immediately is in no wise the heart, nor the brain as a whole, but solely in the innermost part of the brain, viz., a certain very small gland situated in a midway position, and suspended over the passage by which the animal spirits of the anterior cavities communicate with those of the posterior cavities, in such fashion that its slightest movements can greatly alter the course of those spirits; and reciprocally that any change, however slight, taking place in the course of the spirits can greatly change the movements of this gland" (7).

Thus, throughout the long period beginning before the Greeks and including the European Renaissance, the "vital spirits" were viewed as originating outside of the head, distributed throughout the body but altered within the cranium to produce the "psychic pneuma." Yet it is not surprising that this view, clearly stated by Aristotle and Descartes, who based their conclusions on erroneous physiological hypotheses, should have provided the most enduring influences on Western thought. The inference that the life force, the "vital spirits," the soul, was not exclusively engendered within the head, but was contained in all parts of the body, perhaps affirmed a deep intuition and therefore survived despite errors in anatomy.

At all events, the implications of the Galenic physiology of the nervous system remained almost unseen until the early nineteenth century. In the restless creative era of the European Renaissance, there was growing knowledge of the structure of the brain, but still little interest in what it did. A series of energetic and brilliant young Frenchmen contributed vastly to our understanding of its structure but added little to make the brain's significance intelligible.

However, there came a man in the mid-eighteenth century, not French by birth but who worked in France in the atmosphere of growing interest in the nature of man, who dissected the brain. This Franz Josef Gall boldly directed attention to the important facts that the brain was not a cooling device, but was made up of fibers and cells; that its surface was folded to save space; that fibers traversed from one part to the other; and that the rind of the brain functioned, especially in thinking and complex behavior. He claimed that the neural apparatus of speech involved certain portions of the brain rather than others.

Unfortunately, Gall overshot his mark by localizing mental functions too precisely in the brain. He almost wiped out the major significance of his lifework and brought confusion by asserting that specific character qualities were reflected in the size of specific areas of the brain, to be detected not only by inspection of the brain's surface but also by palpation of the skull. This series of specious assumptions led to the elaboration of "phrenology" and to the subsequent rejection by serious students of much that was valuable.

During the nineteenth century, the proponents of the theory of evolution compared the relative size of animal brains to body size and of the separate parts of the brain to the whole brain. Yet, the significance of the relatively large mass of man's cerebral hemispheres to his superior adaptive and intellectual capacities was not seen by many. In the middle of that century, opinions were still divided about the functions of major parts of the brain. Indeed, the brain stem, which constitutes a relatively smaller portion of the human brain and is now known to subserve primitive adaptive capacities, was still the favored site for sensation and consciousness. With the later advent of aseptic surgical techniques, anesthesia, and electrical methods for stimulation of the brain and for recording aspects of its activity, facts could be gathered at least concerning localization of neural equipment for bodily movement. Also, facts about incoming and outgoing neural pathways and the concept of the reflex became common knowledge.

By the end of the nineteenth century, however, the conclusion could no longer be avoided that the cerebral hemispheres of the human brain (the cortex and its adjacent fiber tracts) were the neural apparatus for sensory perception, for learned acts, and for the interpretation of experience. The preoccupation with localization in the brain of such complex functions still remained.

Even up to the middle of the twentieth century, it was erroneously assumed that, since the frontal portion or lobe of a cerebral hemisphere is especially large in man and double the mass of any other lobe, it must be the "center" of the highest mental capacities, such as planning, judgment, restraint, and discrimination. "Wisdom" was allegedly stored in the frontal lobes, "factual knowledge" behind them. However, new data ever more firmly support the sounder concept that for these highest-level functions there is no localization of neural cells in any one part of the cerebral hemispheres.

In the present century, the study of the neuron and its special characteristics has greatly enhanced our knowledge of the anatomy of the nervous system and has offered a means of exploring the way in which input information is dealt with.

THE STEPS FROM NEURONS TO ADAPTIVE BEHAVIOR IN MAN

The neuron is not a fixed entity; indeed it is in perpetual flux of concurrent degradation and renewal. This instability renders it mutable both in adaptive and regressive direction. Far from being set, size goes up or down, varying throughout life. Neurons long deprived of excitation waste away (8) ; conversely, the neuronal nucleus and cell body enlarge in response to excessive excitation (9). Not only its interstices and surfaces but the entire system of the nerve cell are continuously reorganizing. In short, the character and substance of the neuron is significantly altered by its past experience, and furthermore this alteration may persist despite turnover of molecular constituents.

On the irritability of neurons, reflexes can be built. Although there are a few simple reflexes involving only two cells, most reflexes involve an arrangement of at least three cells: one that conveys impulses from the periphery; one or more that connect within the matrix of the nervous system; and one that conveys impulses to a motor or gland cell. All of this is enacted in a fraction of a second, and there is a direct relationship between the input and the output. Complex reflexes are built on simple ones until hundreds of neurons may be involved.

A clue to the way in which a neuron enters into highest level brain function is suggested by its versatility, characteristic irritability, variability, and many connections. The more connections on a nerve cell surface the greater the energy required to keep the system from deteriorating. Energy exchange in a system of neurons requires abundant supplies of oxygenated blood.

To understand the highest integrative functions where there is no direct relationship between input and output, something more complicated than the concept of the reflex is required.

The demonstrable relationship between the highest-level responses and the whole mass of ordered aggregates of neurons in the cerebral hemispheres does give a clue to the nature of the process. Responses are long delayed and are dependent upon countless previous experiences, and variations in the circumstances during stimulation make the output unpredictable. The removal of small amounts of the hemisphere from any region does not abolish the highest-level functions, but it does reduce the capacity for the most complex human activity. It follows as a reasonable assumption that the number and arrangement of nerve cells are of central importance.

In other words, when tremendous numbers of neurons are arranged compactly and in an extremely complex relation to each other, as in the cerebral cortex, especially the neocortex, they acquire through interaction properties quite different from single neurons or those in smaller groups. In this ordered relationship of an enormous number of cells, phenomena arise which are as different from the function of the individual neuron as are the properties of protoplasm from its basic constituents. Of particular relevance to the subject of this essay are the transactions that include the limbic system where stimulation of the brain readily elicits visceral and endocrine effects. The limbic system comprises those structures of the brain that are phylogenetically old, that seem to ring the hylus of the cerebral hemispheres and are thought important for the elaboration and control of emotional life (18). These structures include both cortical and subcortical brain areas, such as the cingulate gyrus, the hippocampus and the amygdaloid complex. Substantial neuronal projections exist to connect these structures with the hypothalamus, where their activity can influence the effector neurons to the pituitary gland and to the viscera. Thus on stimulation of the amygdala, Mason (19) and McHugh and Smith (20) have demonstrated striking adrenocortical effects, Smith and McHugh (21) changes in gastric secretion, Reis and Oliphant (22) changes in heart rate and blood pressure.

The neocortex is the phylogenetically newer portion of the cerebral hemispheres that makes up the bulk of the brain of man and that contains the equipment for the highest level of adaptive behavior. It consists of a thin surface band of cells and a subsurface mass of interlacing fibers. About 7 billion nerve cells are arranged in orderly layers in the cerebral cortex and 70 per cent of their tangential fibers traverse and interconnect in one way or another. The average nerve cell has about 5,000 direct contacts, the larger cells having even more (10). A single nerve cell in the cerebral cortex may receive on its surface several hundred terminals from various other cells and probably the majority of the cortical nerve cells connect directly or indirectly with every cortical field (11). Charles Herrick (12), the distinguished American neuroanatomist, attempted to get some conception of the number of possible connections among these millions of cortical cells. Based on a series of computations, he inferred that there were $10^{2,783,000}$ such connections. To print this number written out in figures would take about two thousand ordinary book pages.

The fact that each neuron may influence many other neurons, some of which are remote, suggest that the "order" of brain tissue is not simply the "checkerboard" order of classical thermodynamics which lacks an extensive dimension but rather is like the "order" of an aperiodic crystal. The huge number of stable interconnecting neural arrangements possible within the brain indicates that the "arrangement density" of the human brain is vastly greater than any analogous physical apparatus suggested to date. Thus, the aspect of brain tissue pertinent to the highest-level functions is not so much location within the hemispheric mass, or connections with peripheral structures, as it is the absolute number of ordered arrangements within the tissue mass.

There are predictably localizable areas for final common

paths in the cortex for incoming and outgoing impulses and sites subserving special functions such as speech. The neural apparatus for motor and sensory function in the hemispheres is quite well localized. Right hand and arm movements result from weak electrical stimulation on the anterior lip of the central sulcus of the cerebral hemisphere on the left side, and left upper extremity movements result from stimulation of a corresponding area on the right side of the brain.

Yet, that the equipment for skilled acts is not sharply limited to one hemisphere is illustrated by the performance of the Hungarian Olympic champion, Takacs. This man represented Hungary in the pistol shooting competition at the Olympics in 1936, holding, at that time, several national and international championships in this sport. In 1938, an accident necessitated amputation of his right arm midway between elbow and wrist. On his discharge from the hospital, Takacs decided to continue competing by shooting with the left hand, which he had never thus used prior to the amputation. The switchover to the left arm was achieved within eight months, and from then on he continued to improve his competence. In 1939, he won the world championship in pistol shooting. He won gold medals in the Olympic games in 1948 and 1952 and in 1956 he entered his fourth Olympic contest (1).

Localization of functions in aggregates of cells so typical of the medulla and mid-brain is not a feature of the highest levels of neural integration. Here, the almost universal interconnection among neurons allows for versatility and particularly for relearning when parts of the brain are damaged. Loss of tissue, however, as it limits the available connections also limits the range and versatility of integrative function. Such limitation correlates far more with the amount than with the localization of brain tissue loss.

While the neural apparatus for the highest level functions of man is in the phylogenetically newer portion of the cerebral hemispheres it has no particular localization therein. Furthermore, in a given individual, removal of a specific amount of the newer portions of these cerebral hemispheres, regardless of site, results in impairment in these highest level functions, grossly proportional to the mass of tissue removed.

In short, the neural apparatus of simple vegetative functions such as eating, elimination, reproduction, the regulation of circulation and content of body fluids, the body temperature, breathing, and other functions involved in keeping the internal environment of the organism in a steady state are concentrated at the base of the brain. These localized aggregates of cells for primitive or lower integrative functions are connected with, and responsive to impulses from the cerebral hemispheres which contain the nerve cells responsible for the highest integrative functions.

In the evolution of the nervous system among vertebrates, the control of reaction patterns, either by initiation or inhibition, moved further and further headward. This is true regardless of whether the reaction pattern is the product of spinal or brain stem integrative devices. In man, therefore, primitive functions have become tied to the newer portion of the cerebral hemispheres and may exhibit themselves under circumstances that seem most inappropriate and remote from the purpose that they mainly serve. The effects of such headward domination, or encephalization, operate in many of man's behavior patterns, usually to his great advantage but sometimes with catastrophic results.

The Nature of the Highest Integrative Functions

Integration, stemming from the Latin, "integrare," "to make whole," has been used here not only to mean the putting together of parts to make a whole but also to imply that the linking of separate functions of the nervous system results in new kinds of functions and not mere combinations of simple elements. Also, it is assumed that intermediate and lower levels of function, activated, inhibited and modulated by higher ones, make their contribution to the synthesis of entirely new functions. In other words, the patterns integrated at spinal and brain-stem levels are dominated by the myriad patterns synthesized at the cortical level, but these are, in turn, integrated not only with each other but also with the effects of stimuli from within and without the central nervous system and with the effects of past experience. This integration in its most elaborate form presumably makes possible those features characteristic of man alone.

Survival for man depends upon his ability to meet new situations. He must have the capacity to endure periods of transition and to persist, return to the task, and recover promptly from the effects of failure, frustration, postponements, and difficult discriminations. These capacities call for a special set of highest integrative functions that supplement learning, recognizing, knowing, remembering, relating and planning. These functions have to do with the maintenance and restoration of organization and serve to restore proper speed of response quickly, lend continuity, and maintain stability during periods of stress. They are subtle, sensitive, and readily impaired. Evidence of their decline are among the first to be noted in deteriorating behavior of human beings.

In the case of damage to the cortex, or loss of tissue whether by surgical removal, injury, infection, or the process of aging, the various categories of highest level functions having to do with the expression of needs, appetites and drives are affected. Fall-off in these functions is manifest in decreased seeking of challenge and adventure, restriction of imagination, lessened human association and exchange, diminished aspiration and striving, abandonment of previously cherished goals, passive acceptance of circumstances, lessened sexual activity, and when the damage is severe, inadequate response to even the minimal requirements of food, shelter and warmth (9, 11).

Second, are those functions having to do with the capacity to respond to symbols as substitutes for biologically significant events, thus employing effectively the mechanisms for goal achievement. These enable the individual to anticipate dangerous or propitious circumstances and to learn, perceive, know, remember, arrange, plan, invent, explore, postpone, modulate and discriminate. Important in this category is the capacity to eliminate responses when they are no longer appropriate.

Third, are those functions that enable man, under circumstances of duress, to integrate elaborate behavior patterns of a defensive or protective nature that are appropriate, adequate, socially acceptable, and sustained.

Fourth, are those functions having to do with the maintenance of organization. These, as mentioned above, serve to lend continuity and maintain stability and proper speed of response and are especially important during periods of stress.

The components of highest integrative functions are not equally fragile. Impairment of speed of response, spontaneity, imagery, creativity, rapid learning, ease of abandoning a pattern when no longer appropriate, capacity for abstraction, and ability to resist the disorganizing effects of stress are evident in subjects with loss of even small amounts of tissue, whereas vocabulary, long utilized skills, behavior patterns, and premorbidly acquired information are not significantly impaired until there is a much greater loss of tissue. With major loss of tissue from the cerebral hemispheres, there is progressive inactivity and finally coma and death.

To recapitulate, the brain functions in general as a unit. Each part is dependent upon the adequate functioning of the remainder, the neocortex, the most recently developed portion of the cerebral hemispheres, serves as the central integrator for over-all adaptation—and adaptation for man must include creating, the ability to withstand changes and threats, the pursuit of adventure, exploration of the new, and, above all, aspiration.

Damage to the human brain stem and neighboring structures alters "consciousness" and impairs the highest integrative functions by depriving the cerebral hemispheres of necessary support. But, assuming proper support from other parts of the body and the lower levels of the nervous system, achieving for man maximum adaptive versatility, is dependent ultimately on the proper functioning of the intact cerebral hemispheres.

THE MECHANISMS IN DISEASE

Granting the ultimate control of the highest integrative functions of the brain over visceral reactions it is interesting to re-examine Claude Bernard's proposition that all disease is the outcome of attempts at adaptation to noxious forces. He suggested that the adaptive response in its intensity, could be more de-structive than the original assaults and that an individual might be damaged gravely through the wrong magnitude of his defensive reaction. For instance, the presence of micro-organisms in the lung evokes cellular and humoral responses that serve to meet invasion and do so effectively. Yet the magnitude of the responses may lead to congestion of the lungs and pneumonia.

Man, with his elaborate brain, is so constituted that he reacts not only to actual assault but to threats and symbols of danger experienced in his past which call forth reactions like those to assault. Also, man's special relation to man introduces another set of factors. Hence, backed by long bedside experience and the realization that much of medicine is the understanding of human motivation, physicians in scattered centers throughout the world have turned their energies into studies of man in his context and the pertinence of this relationship to disease. En-thusiastic about the new wave of interest in purpose and goal, they have become convinced that the scientific method is suitable for such study and can be applied. They are challenged by the opportunity, on the one hand, of keeping medicine compassionate, and, on the other, of making it even more scientific and dynamic.

It is of the first importance for the physician to realize that the spectrum of a man's possible responses to adversity is broad and varied, and that the resultant reaction pattern depends not only on the inherent characteristics of the person and his early experience but also on the characteristics of his environment at the time and his relationship to the people in it, including his physician. The rich variety of reaction to a special kind of stress-ful experience is illustrated by the conduct of prisoners of war especially those exposed to Communist methods of interrogation and indoctrination (13).

This experience is also helpful in pointing up the fact that the concept of disease is not restricted to disordered behavior of the viscera, but includes disturbances in a man's general behavior as well. The widespread deterioration of general be-havior among prisoners has been emphasized and it has become a popular conception that every man has his breaking point (14).

U. N. PRISONERS IN KOREA

Of 6,654 U. S. Army men known to have been in prison camps in the Korean War, all but 463 were taken prisoner in the first twelve months; thus most of the captives were in Communist hands during practically the whole campaign, or almost three years. The management of prisoners during these early days was extremely primitive. During one so-called death march of ninety miles by 500 men, approximately 10 per cent died. Also, during this period atrocities were common. According to official figures, 1,036 Army men were murdered in this way. Word of this spread rapidly through the ranks, and atrocities after capture came to be expected generally.

The knowledge that the North Korean enemy took few prisoners to prison compounds and murdered many of those that fell into their hands was a factor in shaping attitudes of many prisoners when they were actually captured. They were, therefore, especially susceptible to threats of abuse, or death, and were terrified at the prospect of what faced them. This foreknowledge was also a factor in the disorganization that followed contact with the Chinese captors, who not only ordinarily refrained from killing prisoners, but greeted them as friends and instructed them about the "lenient policy." The gist of this "policy" was that prisoners who cooperated with the Communists in their campaign for "international peace" would be dealt with compassionately.

In the final analysis, it is likely that less than two per cent were ever involved in such serious collaborations as writing disloyal tracts or agreeing to spy or to organize for the Communists after the war.

The relatively few collaborators were divided into three categories. The first included those who lacked the stamina to stand even the minimum of discomfort of any kind. The second group were opportunists or those who saw the chance to gain power and prestige through the approval of their captors. The third group, which was very small, were those who became converts to Communism.

Indices used to measure the amounts of pressure applied to the captives were not directly related to the incidence or the type of collaboration. From analysis of a group of American Air Force personnel, for example, it was judged that the harassment applied to those who confessed to participation in germ warfare was not essentially different from that applied to those who did not confess, although there were some obvious differences in the situation within which pressures were applied.

A most telling result of Communist disruptive procedures on United States prisoners of war was the creating in the prisoners of a feeling of being isolated, rejected, or alone. The captors further engendered this feeling of isolation by removing all leaders from among the prisoners. Help for the captives could then only be obtained from the captors. Disease and death are known to follow other kinds of isolation and rejection as in hexing, bone pointing, and excommunications. In experiments with rats in the laboratory, the placing as an interloper of a single strong rat from one organized colony into the midst of relatively weak members of another organized colony would result in rejection and perhaps ultimately in death of the interloper even though physical abuse was minor. Autopsy revealed that the adrenal glands of the dead rats were much enlarged and adrenal secretion depleted. The fact that the interlopers were excluded from the group seemed to make them more vulnerable.

Demoralization, starvation, cold, dysentery, pneumonia, faulty care, and miserable living conditions led to the death of about 38 per cent of the 6,654 U. S. servicemen in captivity during an average period of less than three years. This mortality rate was somewhat higher than that recorded after the forty months of imprisonment of U.S. troops in Japanese prison camps in World War II (about thirty-five per cent). Circumstances in both were dreadful; men were underfed, underclothed, sick, received little medical attention or support from their fellow prisoners or their captors; they were humiliated, abused, and demoralized. In many instances they gave up hope and died.

Categories of Breaking Points

As there is a point of tension at which a rope breaks, a point of breakdown for a swimmer or runner, so there is a "breaking point" for the individual organs and functions of the body, and the regulatory functions of the brain. Military combat is one of the gravest challenges that contemporary man has been called upon to meet, especially as epitomized by the infantryman's experience.

Although it is well known that capacity to endure combat is extremely variable it was possible to ascertain from study of a group of men who had performed well, or even in a distinguished way, that after a given number of days of combat a point is ultimately reached by even the most stalwart, beyond which efficiency falls off seriously. The persons investigated were for the most part highly motivated and reluctant to be relieved of duty, but did ask for reduced responsibility. The need to remain alert, the lack of comfort, and combat noises, especially at night, evoked in these combat-sensitized soldiers a depleting "on guard" reaction. They were excessively tremulous, sweated profusely, complained of dyspepsia, were extremely cautious, had difficulty making decisions, avoided responsibilities, and said they would soon be killed in battle.

The breaking point of the average man in the Army of the United States was reached after about eighty-five days of combat. Indeed, 75 per cent could be expected to have broken down by combat day 140 and 90 per cent by combat day 210.

Loss of sleep was probably a significant factor in such collapse. The almost continuous shelling, the strange night noises, flares, sentry and patrol duties, rain, snow, cold, heat, insects, and the ever-present threat of the enemy—conspired to make sleep at best intermittent and scanty. In spite of his lack of sleep, the soldier had to undergo long periods of exertion, more often than not on a diet that was deficient in calories. Even when food was available, he either would not carry enough of it with him, or he was too frightened to eat the proper amount.

After sufficient exposure to the circumstances of battle, requiring accurate and appropriate gunfire and other aggressive actions—marching, integrating with the maneuvers of others, recognizing and interpreting complicated signals, bearing heavy burdens, withstanding high or low temperatures and bodily injury—disorganized and delayed performance may be expected. In this sense, every man has a "breaking point." This breaking point is postponed by means of special training or particular supports that engender "fitness" in particular ways. There is no way to engender "fitness" in all spheres. The postponement of "breaking point" is always in terms of a particular job, task, and integrated aggressive or defensive action.

Commitment may be viewed as a form of adaptive behavior evoked in response to situations which an individual perceives as challenging or threatening to his concept of himself as a man, or to the very survival of his tribe. Hence to be committed implies the maintenance of a belief, faith, conviction; adherence to a course of action; persistence in pursuit of a goal; remaining loyal to persons, party, team, gang, platoon, regiment, and country; and being steadfast to one's values. Furthermore, it implies such persistence, adherence, loyalty, and steadfastness in the face of obstacles, deprivations, bodily and mental defects, and even death. Highly developed commitment is found in relatively few persons.

Acts which humiliate, destroy self-esteem, create feelings of being isolated, rejected, abandoned or unwanted may impair integrative capacity at the highest level. Threats of punishments by beating, threats of harm to loved ones, or falsehoods about the state of one's associates, family or country, may be damaging. Likewise, a host of deprivations and denial of sleep, as well as exhaustion, pain, starvation, malnutrition, sepsis and intoxication affect integrative capacity in most men but do not cause breach of faith in those who are committed.

SLEEP DEPRIVATION AND PRIMARY PURPOSE

Sleep deprivation carried to a point of induced stupor failed to evoke false confessions from committed flyers who were prisoners of war in Korea (14) .

A few years ago in civil circumstances, a man had an opportunity to further the cause of the care of ill children and to contribute to scientific knowledge by proving that he could remain awake 200 hours (15-17) . His motivation was fortified by public interest and approval. This experiment was done with widespread publicity which he hoped would also help his own career as a radio and television broadcaster. During the eight-day period, entirely deprived of sleep, it was necessary for him to broadcast his three-hour program and make one television appearance daily. He was keenly sensitive to the dangers for his performance of inappropriate remarks or behavior, and carelessness about timing. Careful studies made in the laboratory during this period showed progressive, grave impairment of his capacity to learn, attend, remember, concentrate, and discriminate. Moreover, in the laboratory between broadcasts, he became suspicious, profane, obscene, impulsive, bold, explosive, and truculent, and had delusions of being poisoned and that those about him were part of a plot to ruin his career. Most of the time his speech was mumbling and slow as were all his movements. Yet, his performance of his task as a broadcaster, involving previously acquired skills, and on which his ambition was focused, was articulate and professional. Though he lacked his usual sparkle, he was not careless, profane, or indiscreet in his broadcasts, even at the end of this long period of sleep deprivation, when truly many of his highest-level functions had long passed the "breaking point."

In summary, when the brain is damaged either through surgical means, through actions of poisons, or by distorting an individual's interaction with his environment, perceptions may be blurred and mental processes may be slowed. Recent memory becomes faulty, thinking becomes difficult, and if pressed, some individuals may develop fantasies, hallucinations, and they may follow suggestions too readily. The results may throw subjects into panic. Similarly, in hypnosis, the subject becomes suggestible and often, as a result, his behavior becomes bizarre. But, it is impossible to induce him to do an act which is strongly opposed to his convictions. Persons with major amounts of brain loss or damage who have impaired functions that make them incapable of many of their skills, may hold on to a faith. As long as he is conscious, a man is capable of remaining committed to basic beliefs and convictions, although in many ways his behavior may deteriorate.

A study of a few of the survivors of prisoner of war camps who have since become unusually effective citizens is significant.

Despite exposure to many stressful conditions, the imprisonment for them was a painful but temporary interruption in a life viewed as a continuum. They were convinced that they would not be imprisoned long. They were able to extract a few satisfactions even while enduring deprivations. New interests were cultivated (one man raised rabbits for food and began breeding them for increased size). Mind and spirit were mainly focused on life as it was to be lived into the future. The immediate distress seemed less real; the future more substantial. Plans were made for occupation, marriage, family, children, often with meticulous and obsessive detail, including domicile, city or town, education for self and kin, entertainment, the kind of food and where it would be eaten. Among these prisoners academic courses were organized, teaching carried out, seminars and discussions led. These men formed tightly knit groups, believed in, helped each other, and even laughed together. Immediately after liberation, a few had transient illnesses, but there is little to indicate that their vitality had been sapped. Indeed, some have assumed major responsibilities.

Although apparently atavistic processes (adaptations) are aroused by situations that are threatening to the individual, the resultant need not be disease, disability, tissue damage, and death. The inherent versatility of the integrative process allows for modifications or for learning new adaptations, or indeed in certain crisis situations, the organism without time for learning may call into being an adaptive reaction which was heretofore undreamed of and which saves him from destruction. The mechanisms whereby the myriad alternate possibilities are selected are not understood at present. It is clear on the input side that when a threat is accompanied by information to the effect that the environment is supportive, and when the integrative process includes the play of self confidence and satisfying purpose the resultant bodily manifestations are more likely to be constructive than destructive.

BIBLIOGRAPHY

1. WOLFF, H. G.: The mind-body relationship. In: *An Outline of Man's Knowledge.* New York, Doubleday, 1960, Chap. 2, pp. 43-72.

2. CHAPMAN, L., and WOLFF, H. G.: The cerebral hemispheres and the highest integrative functions of man. *Arch. Neurol., I:*357-424, 1959.

3. ONIANS, R. B.: *The Origins of European Thought about the Body, the Mind, the Soul, the World, Time and Fate.* Cambridge Univ. Press, 1951.

4. REEVES, JOAN WYNNE: *Body and Mind in Western Thought.* Pelican Psychology Series—A Penguin Book. Glasgow Press, 1958.

5. POYNTER, F. N. L.: *Editor: The History and Philosophy of Knowledge of the Human Brain.* Oxford, England, Blackwell, 1959.

6. ARISTOTLE: *The Works of Aristotle,* W. D. Roos, Ed. Oxford, Clarendon Press, 1931.

7. DESCARTES, RENE: *Les Passions de l'Ame.* Article 31 in Descartes *Philosophical Writings,* Trans. by Norman Kemp Smith. London, MacMillan, 1952.

8. YOUNG, I. J.: Histologic and histochemical alterations in isolated spinal cord segment. (To be published.)

9. CHAPMAN, LORING F. and WOLFF, HAROLD G.: The cerebral hemispheres and the highest integrative functions of man. *Arch. Neurol., 1:*357-424, 1959.

10. YOUNG, J. Z.: *A Model of the Brain.* London, Oxford University Press, 1964.

11. SHOLL, D. A.: *The Organization of the Cerebral Cortex.* London, Methuen, 1956.

12. HERRICK, C. J.: *The Evolution of Human Nature.* Austin, Univ. Texas Press, 1956.

13. HINKLE, L. E., and WOLFF, H. G.: Communist interrogation and indoctrination of "enemies of the state." Analysis of methods used by the Communist State Police (A Special Report). *Arch. Neurol. Psychiat., 76:*115-174, 1956.

14. WOLFF, H. G.: Every man has his breaking point—(?) The conduct of prisoners of war. *Milit. Med., 125:*85-104, 1960.

15. WEST, L. J.: Psychiatry, "Brain washing" and the American character. *Amer. J. Psychiat., 120:*842, 1964.

16. WEST, L. J.: Psychopathology produced by sleep deprivation. Ass. Res. Nerv. and Ment. Dis., *Sleep and Altered States of Consciousness* In Press.

17. WOLFF, H. G.: Unpublished observations with L. J. West.
18. MCLEAN, P. D.: Psychosomatics. Chapter in: *Handbook of Physiology: Neurophysiology*, Vol. III, 1960, Chapter 69., pp. 1723-1744.
19. MASON, J. W.: Plasma 17-hydroxycorticosteroid levels during electrical stimulation of the amygdaloid complex in conscious monkeys. *Am. J. Physiology, 196*:44-48, 1959.
20. MCHUGH, P. D. and SMITH, G. P.: Brain stimulation and plasma 17-hydroxycorticosteroid control. *Physiologist, 7*:204, 1964.
21. SMITH, G. P. and MCHUGH, P. R.: Gastric secretory response to amygdaloid stimulation. *Physiologist, 7*:259, 1964.
22. REIS, D. J. and OLIPHANT, M. C.: Bradycardia and tachycardia following electrical stimulation of the amygdaloid region in monkeys. *J. Neurophysiology, 27*:893-912, 1964.

Chapter VI

PATTERNS OF SOCIAL ADJUSTMENT
AND DISEASE

I<small>T IS INTERESTING</small> that the word "threat" derives from an old English root which also yielded the word "throng," thus suggesting the potentially noxious nature of social relationships. Indeed, two individuals living in relative tranquility may, because of some social upheaval not even directly involving either of them, become enemies (1).

It is helpful to consider the individual as a living system entirely dependent upon maintaining a satisfactory relationship with his total environment. A man's life is dependent upon his ability to maintain a satisfactory body temperature; a satisfactory intake of food, fluids and air; a satisfactory elimination of waste products, and a satisfactory amount of rest and activity. It is equally necessary for him to maintain a satisfactory relationship with the other human beings in his environment, and especially with those humans who by kinship or long association have acquired a special meaning to him (2).

When any of these necessary relationships between man and his environment are disturbed, there develop within him feelings which are unpleasant, and stimulate him to take whatever action is necessary to bring them to an end. There may be such unpleasant feelings as anxiety, fear, anger, loneliness, sadness, and dejection, which arise out of disturbed relations to the total environment and the people in it. When beset by these feelings, there are other unpleasant sensations of hunger, thirst, fatigue, sleeplessness, excessive warmth, or coldness, and all sorts of pain. These sensations originate within the human body as a result of disturbances of body processes.

Even minor and transient social disruptions were associated with measurable physiological changes in patients undergoing metabolic balance studies on a research ward (3-6). The patients, living together in relatively close confinement, were being investigated with respect to their day-to-day life experiences and emotional reactions by observers who had no knowledge of the metabolic data. Of 213 patient-days on which suitable balance data were available, 146 were judged as non-stressful and sixty-seven as being stressful. In forty-eight or 72 per cent of the incidents, significant deviations from a control period in Na, P, Ca, and N balance occurred. When the stressful incidents were segregated as to whether the general atmosphere of the ward at the time was troubled or tranquil, 86 per cent of incidents occurring during a troubled period of minor social upheaval were associated with metabolic deviations while during periods of tranquility on the ward, only 48 per cent of stressful incidents were accompanied by significant alterations in the metabolic indicators. Significant deviations in metabolic balance were noted on less than 10 per cent of days separately judged as non-stressful.

Important adjustments to cultural and social pressures and to interpersonal stresses are made through the interpretive areas of the brain (7). Sechenov, who had worked with Claude Bernard, was impressed not so much by the constancy of the *milieu intereure* as by its capacity to adapt, presumably under nervous control, to changes in the *milieu extereure* (8, 9).

It is often the threat of disruption of established relationships which may call forth pernicious adaptive reactions and disease. Nearly twenty-five centuries ago, Hippocrates (10) reminded his contemporaries of the risk of such changes when he said: "Those things which one has been accustomed to for a long time, although worse than things which one is not accustomed to, usually give less disturbance." Even in host parasite relationships there are illuminating examples of the noxious nature of change.

There is a group of virus organisms that, because of their long continued relation with laboratory mice, cease to precipitate infection in mice except under very special circumstances. This equilibrium has been reached through generations of exposure of mouse and virus to each other under laboratory conditions. The end result is that newly born mice are already infected in utero and harbor the virus in a latent form in their tissues for the remainder of their lives. Among such may be mentioned the pneumonia virus, the virus of lymphocytic choriomeningitis (11, 12), the gray lung virus (13) and the pneumonitis virus (14, 15). A feature of the relations of these microorganisms to their mouse hosts is that minimal changes in the airways, such as result from intranasal injection of physiological saline solution, broth, or serum, may precipitate serious pneumonitis.

Objection might be raised to these examples, inasmuch as they are products of the laboratory. Yet, comparable reactions occur under non-laboratory conditions. The first of these has to do with parakeets (16). In Texas, Florida and California there are large aviaries that breed these birds for commercial purposes. From time to time, the bird colonies have epidemics of psittacosis, and usually after a sufficient period the epidemics die down and for a time the community is free of the infection. The micro-organism remains latent in the tissue of the surviving birds. This desirable state may be hastened by separating the sexes. For example, in a colony of 2,000 parakeets, shortly after the separa-tion of the sexes, active psittacosis disappeared. However, within five or six weeks of the time the sexes were brought together again with breeding and egg laying, a new epidemic exhibited itself. Hence, what seems like a propitious circumstance, namely, that of bringing the sexes together, is followed by catastrophe for the colony involved. Certainly, the mating and egg laying which precipitate the epidemic are not, in themselves, morbid or noxious forces. The crowding and competition which the change induced may be. Rahe and Holmes have recently docu-mented a close relationship between the number of major social changes, favorable or unfavorable, and the occurrence of disease states in humans (117).

An extremely dramatic instance of change precipitating in-fectious disease is seen in the role of the seasons in the epi-demiology of swine influenza. Swine influenza results from the activation of a latent virus, in this instance, living in the lung worm of the pig (Shope, 1943) (17). Under ordinary circum-stances, the lung worm and its affiliate virus cause no disease or untoward manifestation. A certain number of embryonated ova from the lung worm pass into the gut of the pig and are excreted.

These are ingested by the earthworm where the lung worm lives out part of its life cycle. Ultimately, the earthworm and its contained lung worm and swine influenza virus are ingested by a second pig which then, in turn, harbors the lung worm and the virus in its own lung. All of these steps are accomplished without morbid manifestations. In the summer, this established equilibrium is not easily disturbed but in late October and November a variety of non-specific agents can disturb the equilibrium. So benign a procedure as inoculation of the pig with a *Hemophilus influenza suis* in itself of little pathological significance may precipitate severe influenzal infection. In short, a vague, ill-defined factor, the changing season, disturbs the relationship between two living forms and activates an infection which may be lethal.

Herpes simplex and rabies infections represent latency of viruses in man.

Herpes simplex is a classical example of a latent virus infection. The virus is dormant in the majority of human beings and there are many flaring factors which may provoke the virus to appear. Koprowski (18), lists them as fever (induced or due to infection), cold, menstruation, exposure to sun, and, last but not least, emotional upset. Intensive study of a group of ten patients (19) who had repeated attacks of herpes simplex at frequent intervals without any apparent cause were revealed to share similar reaction patterns involving anxiety, frustration, shame and guilt. Appropriate psychotherapy achieved relief of symptoms which was sustained for many months. Two independent groups of investigators (20, 21) have induced recurrent activation of herpes simplex infection by suggestion during hypnosis. Kowprowski has also suggested that similar flaring factors may be associated with shorter incubation periods and perhaps the precipitation of an attack of rabies in an exposed individual.

There is much to indicate that pituitary and adrenal endocrine mechanisms are involved in regulating higher mammals' adjustments to change and threats. Thus, immunologic mechanisms are suppressed by hormones of the adrenal cortex. The suppression of defense mechanisms against infection by the increased amount of circulating corticosteroid hormones may explain in part increased susceptibility to infection during exposure to cold, surgical trauma or emotionally troublesome life situations. The introduction of cortisone into an animal may so alter an established equilibrium between rat and parasite that such diverse microbial forms as viruses, plasmodia and bacilli become viable. Thus, numerous virus forms in mice and the polio virus in hamsters are far more invasive after the administration of cortisone to the host. For example, Schwartzman (22) has shown that polio virus injected intracerebrally, ordinarily resulting in a mortality of 27 per cent in hamsters, can, after the injection of cortisone, result in a mortality of 100 per cent. Studies with malaria plasmodia similarly showed that cortisone increased the severity of the infectious state. The provocative studies of Dubos and others show analagous effects with tuberculosis. These data suggest a mechanism for the morbid process set in motion during periods of adaptation (23).

Again, the formulation of Dubos epitomizes in general terms what has been suggested by these data:

"All living things, from men to the smallest microbe, live in association with other living things. Through the phenomena of biological evolution, an equilibrium is established which permits the different components of biological systems to live at peace together, indeed often to help one another. Whenever the equilibrium is disturbed by any means whatever, either internal or external, one of the components of the system is favored at the expense of the other . . . and then come about the processes of disease" (24).

Also, according to Sigerist (25):

". . . In every epoch certain diseases are in the foreground and . . . are characteristic of this epoch and fit into its whole structure. It seems as though the powers that ordain the style for and stamp their impress upon a certain epoch affect even disease.

"The Middle Ages, for instance, were dominated by disease of the common people—such as the plague, leprosy, and the epidemic neuroses—which appeared in the sixth to the fourteenth centuries, thus outlining that period in history. In the Renaissance it was syphilis, a distinctly individualistic disease, to which no one is subject but which is acquired through a volitional act.

"In the discordant Baroque era the foreground is occupied by diseases which might be called deficiency diseases like camp-fever, scurvy and ergotism on the one hand and on the other by diseases which might be called luxury diseases like gout, dropsy and hypochondriasis. Tuberculosis of the lungs, chlorosis and similar diseases are pathological expressions of the romantic period, while the nineteenth century, with its tremendously increased industrialization, the development of great cities and the accelerated life tempo, brought about industrial diseases, general nervousness and neuroses of many kinds."

High mortality from tuberculosis associated with increased industrialization persisted throughout the nineteenth and early twentieth centuries during migrations from rural to urban life and from one country to another (26). The high mortality has usually been considered the result of exposure to cold and rain, lack of food, excessive effort, crowding, and contact of a migratory population with new and fresh sources of infections to which they had developed insufficient immunity. However, the explanation is not a simple one. In a given society, mortality from tuberculosis reaches its peak within ten to twenty years after industrialization and thereafter falls off rapidly (27-31).

The decline in mortality from tuberculosis in England and in the U.S.A. particularly in Massachusetts parallel each other and began shortly after 1850. These communities were industrialized at about the same time (1830-1850). In contrast, in nations and communities such as Ireland, the northern part of Sweden, Japan and Chile, where industrialization began far later, the peak and the decline occur correspondingly later. Indeed, in Chile, the last of the group to be industrialized, the peak has not yet been reached.

Also, major crises in national life are associated with a marked rise in mortality from tuberculosis. When the mortality curves of the state of Prussia are followed from the last quarter of the nineteenth century, it is seen that the curve is steadily downgrade until 1914. Then, with the onset of World War I and perhaps even preceding it, the shape of the curve changes until it rises rapidly and reaches a new peak in 1918. It promptly declines again thereafter and continues its downward course even through the early 1920's, despite serious food shortage in

Prussia during this period. It rises again in 1923 during a period of serious economic inflation, and falls off thereafter (32).

It could be postulated that such a rise in incidence of a disease in nations at war is directly related to combat, bombing and battle conditions, since England, Austria and Italy exhibited similar peaks in mortality between 1914 and 1918; but since the Netherlands and Sweden also demonstrated rises between 1914 and 1918, combat circumstances as such cannot be the main factors. Augmented industrialization, urbanization, population dislocations, internal and external migrations and the disorganization of family life as well as other changes that accompany such basic social reorganization as occurred throughout Europe during the first World War, do not allow isolation of a single most relevant factor. The inference is that a crisis or calamity that imposes change major and rapid enough to disorganize the way of life of the individuals in a nation may diminish the individual's resistance to microorganisms. This is in keeping with bedside experience, since it has long been recognized that situations which the individual perceives as adverse are pertinent to the onset and exacerbation of tuberculosis (28, 29).

As mentioned above, deaths from tuberculosis have decreased steadily in Massachusetts since 1853, though without conspicuous change in rate after introduction of important public health measures until the introduction of effective antibiotics. The tuberculosis infection rate, as indicated by x-ray and sensitivity tests, is still not remarkably reduced. It is thus quite evident that infection is in itself insufficient to induce high mortality. Since the 1850's in the U.S.A., mortality from other infections besides tuberculosis has declined, as, for example, from pneumococcus pneumonia (30, 31).

When a sizable block of Ireland's population emigrated to American seacoast cities, they were better fed and had more promise for the future. Yet the death rate from tuberculosis among the Irish in New York City, for instance, was one hundred per cent greater than at the same time in Dublin (33, 34).

That "industrialization" is not per se the sole lethal ingredient in the alterations of the individual's relations to his environment is shown by the fact that a greater number of

American Indians died from tuberculosis when they were moved from the plains to reservations, in miles not very far distant and where sanitation was better (35). Tuberculosis killed hordes of Bantu natives who had been moved from the country outside of Johannesburg into the environs of the city (27). When told that they were about to die, some asked to be sent back to their kraals. Many died, a few survived, but tuberculosis was widely spread by them in the native village. Interestingly enough, deaths from tuberculosis did not vastly increase with the spread of the disease, suggesting that the Bantus in their native environment could deal better with the infection.

The view that pulmonary tuberculosis is often activated in adults in a setting of life crisis is supported by the results of intensive studies of two small groups of personnel in a hospital for pulmonary disease, both very much exposed to tuberculosis from patients with active disease. Both groups had a professional attitude about the hazards and took the usual precautions against infection. The ones who became ill with active tuberculosis were those who felt severely threatened by personal events in their lives. Those who remained well had little or no sense of being threatened by circumstances (36).

Another aspect of increasing morbidity and mortality during a period of readaptation associated with a radical change in environment is that exhibited by epidemics of meningoccus meningitis that occurred with the onset of barrack life in the United States Army. The rise in the "carrier" rate with the intimacy of barrack life is but one aspect of the widespread changes in environment and the demands for adjustment made upon a large dislocated male population during periods of war (37).

Dubos has demonstrated that the capacity of the tuberculosis organism to multiply is affected by factors other than major reduction in the defensive immunologic and antibody mechanisms. Minor changes in the acid-base balance in the environment of the micro-organism can determine whether it flourishes or is held in an arrested state. Such relatively minor changes could occur under stressful circumstances and during readjustments in a new environment. Thus, susceptibility to infection is not always related only to immune bodies in the blood, but to local changes in tissues as well. In this connection, although increased adrenocortical secretion occurring under stress may, as pointed out earlier, suppress immunologic mechanisms, it is interesting that Bakke *et al.*, found that the change in the titer of certain specific antibodies in the blood during fluctuations in stress and strain are minimal (38).

THE RELATION OF ENVIRONMENT TO PATHOGENICITY OF ORGANISMS

A dramatic example of the effect of environmental factors in promoting one proclivity to the relative exclusion of many others is afforded by the experiments of Dubos (39). When the micro-organism (bacillus S III) which decomposes the capsular polysaccharide of Type III pneumococcus was placed in a casein hydrolysate medium, no appreciable amount of polysaccharide-decomposing enzyme was elaborated. But, when these same organisms were resuspended in a solution of polysaccharide, production of enzyme was conspicuous.

The rapid development of the specific enzyme activity in the presence of the polysaccharide suggested that the cells recovered from the casein hydrolysate culture possessed a "latent" form of the enzyme which became "activated" in the presence of the specific substrate. The specific enzyme produced by the S III bacillus belongs to the group of "adaptive" enzymes (39) which are formed only as a response to the specific substrate.

The implication of these observations clearly is that major alterations in an organism, perhaps as an epiphenomenon of adaptation, can be induced by a specific cultural component.

Observations of this kind, of which there are many, led Rene Dubos to conclude, "There is reason to wonder whether any microorganism cannot become the cause of disease if suitable conditions are provided for it. Thus, there are many circumstances, some of which are of common occurrence in human medicine, where the physical, chemical, physiological, and probably *psychological* factors which affect the host play far more decisive parts in the causation of disease than does the presence of this or that microorganism."

SOCIAL CHALLENGES FOR MAN

The challenges of routine daily life especially those relating to one's standing in relation to his fellows may weigh heavily in the balance toward health or disease.

Among his strongest drives is man's need to be part of a group. The pressures and goals defined by his culture do much to further or to block his inherent and deep-rooted individual potentialities. In a study reported by Christenson and Hinkle (40), 139 managerial employees in a corporation having the same average salaries and working in comparable environments were divided into two groups, C and H, and studied for one year. Both groups ranged in age from twenty-two to thirty-one years, with but little difference in average ages. In Group C were fifty-five fairly recent college graduates who had been hired as managers, in many instances directly from college. In Group H were eighty-four high school graduates who had risen from the ranks to attain their managerial positions. The two groups of men were compared in terms of the relative amount and kind of illness experienced by the individual members. The Group H men experienced more new illnesses of many kinds during the period of observation. They also had a significantly greater number of chronic illnesses: more acne, more constipation, more vasomotor rhinitis, more dental caries, as well as more instances of arthritis, bronchitis, and symptoms of anxiety and tension. They had more impairments resulting from previous diseases: more scars, more absent teeth, more asymptomatic hemorrhoids. The "risk of death" estimated from actuarial tables containing physical characteristics known to be statistically predictive of longevity, small as it was, was nevertheless ten times higher in H group of men than among the C's.

The H group men displayed more of those signs which are commonly considered to be prognostic of later cardiovascular disease. More of them had blood pressure higher than 140 mm Hg systolic or 90 diastolic on readings obtained under standard conditions. More of them were overweight, more of them had depression of T-waves and ST segments in precordial leads, as observed in the electrocardiogram, and more of them had early evidence of arteriosclerosis in the eye grounds.

Measures of heredity between the two groups showed no essential differences. So far as could be ascertained diets were similar, although eating habits differed, in that the H group ate smaller breakfasts and ate more between meals. They also smoked more.

Despite the similarity of the two groups in their present job characteristics and their present physical and social environments, notable differences existed in past experiences and present life situations. The Group H men had come from larger families having more ill members, and many had worked during adolescence to help support themselves and their siblings. Practically all of the Group H men had worked as blue collar laborers for a number of years after high school graduation before attaining their present managerial positions. Even during the one year period of observation, the Group H men appeared to have presented to them more challenges, threats and demands than did the Group C men. They had married earlier and had more dependents. They had more domestic, financial and interpersonal difficulties. Some had extra jobs, many were taking vocational training and some were attending college at night. Thus at the cost of exposure to a greater quantity and variety of challenges the Group H subjects were "getting ahead in the world" while the Group C subjects could be said from a social point of view merely to be continuing at the level from which they had started.

In another study, the prevalence of a large variety of illnesses in relation to life experiences and social adjustment was examined among 3,500 ostensibly healthy men and women. These included not only native Americans but also an homogeneous group of foreign-born persons with an entirely different cultural tradition. Several striking generalizations came from these studies.

Illness was not spread evenly throughout the population. In fact, about one-quarter of the individuals accounted for more than one-half the episodes of illness. There were more than twenty times as many episodes of illness in the least healthy members of the group as there were in the most healthy members. Some of the latter individuals had as little as twenty days of absence from work because of illness in twenty years, whereas some of the least healthy ones had more than 1,300 days in the same length of time.

The persons with the most illness also had the widest variety of illnesses. Indeed, it was rare to find an individual with much illness who had disease confined to one category. It should be emphasized that the distribution of illness in the population was not random. Those with a great deal of illness had not only many minor but also numerous major disorders of a medical, surgical, and psychiatric nature, including infections, injuries, new growth, and serious disturbances in mood, thought, and behavior.

The episodes of illness clustered; that is, there were many episodes in one or more particular years, contiguous with other periods during which few or no illnesses occurred.

When the healthiest group was compared with the group most frequently ill, yet not chronically ill, it became evident that physical hardships, geographic dislocation, exposure to infection, rapid social change, and interpersonal problems occurred with almost equal frequency in both groups.

There were, however, striking differences in the two groups. Those most often ill, in contrast to those least often ill, viewed their lives as having been difficult and unsatisfactory. They were more inflexibly oriented toward goals, duties, and responsibilities. They reacted sharply to events that confronted them. Typically, they were in conflict about pursuing their own ends and ambitions on the one hand and on the other acting responsibly and according to early learned principles toward wives, children, parents and friends. They were "concerned" people who "took things seriously" and many were ambitious and had worked hard to "get ahead" in the world. Most of them were very much aware of their emotional difficulties and their poor adjustment in interpersonal relations, and many complained about them. They were more anxious, self-absorbed, "turned-in," unduly sensitive people who sought much support and encouragement.

In contrast, those who were least often ill viewed their lives as having been relatively satisfactory. They came of more stable and complete families, capable of and willing to lend more support. They viewed themselves as having had preferred sibling positions, good marriages, and rewarding careers. They were convinced that the relations between their parents were good as were their relations to their parents. They exhibited an unusual lack of concern when confronted by situations that a neutral observer would consider threatening. They were as a group more outgoing and more resilient. They evaluated impersonal events objectively, were less anxious, and had fewer morbid fears. They were able to rationalize, deny, and convert their attitudes and feelings from hostility to concern without undue cost to themselves. They avoided becoming involved in the problems of others, "took things less seriously," had experienced little inner conflict, and their interpersonal relations were easy and satisfactory. They were not aware of nor did they show evidence of having disturbing emotional reactions.

Further evidence of the salubrious effects of emotional support from the family and community derive from the study of Roseto, Pennsylvania. A strikingly low death rate from myocardial infarction was correlated with a cohesive and mutually supporting family and community structure. Lack of emotional nourishment from relationships with fellow men may have grave consequences (41, 42, 119, 120, 121).

Social Taboos

It is apparent from anthropological studies that certain attitudes engendered by society have among their purposes the creation of feelings of rejection, ostracism and social isolation. These have to do with the maintenance of established order in the tribe and can be operated for policing and controlling individuals. In primitive societies, such means as black magic, bone pointing and pouri-pouri are used to engender in man fear and feelings of being abandoned through which, in its extreme form, an authoritative member of the tribe can bring about death. That deaths do occur has been authenticated, although the mode of death is unclear.

Walter B. Cannon, in 1942 (43), reviewed the evidence on the mechanism of death by magic and suggested at the time that the individuals died because of a state of sustained fear and shock, coupled with stoppage of food and fluid.

An informative instance was observed during World War II in a native of a small island near New Guinea (44). The subject exhibited at no time the tachycardia, the cold, clamy skin and the hypotension characteristic of shock, except perhaps during the terminal moments. In common with those others who died in this manner, the victim had an awareness that he was considered as dead by his tribe. On being ignored, excommunicated and rejected, and after a period of panic, he became listless, immobile, apathetic and inert. He expressed at no time a desire to live and acted as though convinced that his end was inevitable. He, like others, took to his pallet, refused food and water, and died in nine days.

The subject was observed in the Southwest Pacific, on Goodenough Island, d'Entrecasteaux Group, British New Guinea. He was approximately thirty years old, and in the Australian Regimental Hospital under the care of Sgt. Hill of the Australian military service. The patient was admitted with the complaint that "pouri pouri" had been made "against" him, indicating that a potion had been mixed and incantations recited by a competent person. The subject had been made aware that he was a victim of "pouri-pouri;" the implication was that he had broken a taboo. The tribe treated him as though he were excommunicated and no longer one of them, chiefly by neglecting, ignoring and avoiding him.

The examination on admission revealed an individual who looked older than his estimated chronological age, but not much older than others of his tribe of comparable age. He exhibited splenomegaly, skin yaws, and slight arterial hypertension. Although he did not appear severely ill, his state varied between one of frank depression and apathy, but not one of terror. He was silent, remained inert on his pallet, refused to eat and drank no water or fluids. His pulse rate was 65, his heart was somewhat enlarged and x rays of his chest were not contributory. His blood pressure subsequently was within normal range or slightly elevated. His past history revealed that he probably had had malaria, dysentery and yaws. He showed no interest in the attention of the physicians. A successful attempt was made to get an anti-potion from his tribe and this was brought to his bedside with the assurance that his health would return. For a short time, he partook slightly of the mixture of materials presented to him, but then rejected it. The anti-potion then remained at his side, untouched. He became increasingly apathetic, seemed detached and resigned; he barely moved; his bed covers lay undisturbed for hours. His skin and mouth were dry. His urine contained a slight amount of albumin and had a high specific gravity. He was not seen to pass excreta after the first few days. He received penicillin, arsenicals and digitalis. No one came to see him and he interested himself in no way in other patients. He was found dead in bed on the ninth day after admission. Autopsy revealed cirrhosis of the liver, splenomegaly and widespread arteriosclerosis. Also, amyloidosis of the spleen, kidneys, pancreas and liver was revealed on histological examination. No immediate cause of death was discovered. The likelihood is that the death was one of suicide due to voluntary rejection of fluids. As such it falls into the general category of self-murder brought about by tribal rejection.

Sainsbury has shown that the high incidence of suicide in certain regions of London can be related to the number of rooming houses and hotels where persons living alone become convinced of their isolation and rejection (45). In a community that is mobile, human relationships are perfunctory, and those values and standards are lacking by which it controls its members, and by which they order their lives; suicide is more likely among individuals thus socially isolated. Suicide in our own society, ranking in some states of the United States as the fifth commonest cause of death in adults, exhibits high rates in less populous states where people live far apart from others (46). It is in many instances the sequel of a similar conviction of isolation on the part of the individual involved.

RAPID SOCIAL CHANGE

Not only may isolation from social institutions designed to regulate behavior engender in persons a feeling of having lost support, or of being set adrift from safe moorings, but so may radical changes in social patterns that occur in so-called rapidly developing societies.

In Central India, where a society is undergoing rapid cultural change, it is alleged that diarrhea, ulcerative colitis, neurocirculatory asthenia and asthma are far more common among the relatively opulent, well-nourished, hygienically oriented, educated, so-called Westernized Indians of the large communities than among the ignorant, unschooled, unhygienic, highly religious and often overworked, underfed, non-Westernized people of small villages (47). The former are adjusting themselves to a new set of values and are caught between two systems, finding little support in either. Among these are outwardly bland, but inwardly striving, dissatisfied, tense, anxious and hostile persons who exhibit offensive and defensive protective patterns. In our culture, the protective symptoms mentioned are commonly found in essentially passive, nonparticipating persons who have been made angry by situations that they cannot or do not face.

C. A. Seguin (48), after more than ten years' observation of manual workers treated in the Social Security program's hospital in Lima, Peru, reported (1956) on *The Psychosomatic Maladjustment Syndrome* which incapacitates great numbers of laborers who have migrated from their small, primitive agricultural communities in the sierras to the coastal cities, principally Lima. Impelled by (1) economic stringency (family growth debars earning a livelihood on impoverished, poorly-worked land); (2) ambition (a worker on the coast is paid ten times as much as one in the highlands), and (3) fascination with the lure of the sophisticated life in the metropolitan centers, over 150,000 mostly young men and women flock annually to the coast, increasing the population of Lima alone by 54 per cent since 1940.

Seguin accounts for their "terrible" difficulties in adaptation, which cause so many to become ill from such a sudden, drastic change in their way of living, as follows: the highlanders not only come from a totally different climate and landscape, but also, being mostly Indians, are physiologically and linguistically a race apart from the largely Negro, Asiatic European mixtures of the coast. Their early conditioning in closely-united family groups, engaged in simple, individualistic contact with the land, has made them biologically alien to the urban, industrialized proletariat in which family life is almost non-existent. In addition, the strangeness of their new type of work, food, and eating habits is profoundly unsettling. In many cases, the newcomer, ambitious and desirous to progress from his lower-class status, tries to study at night after working all day—an effort which further complicates his adaptation. The time elapsing between the arrival in Lima and the appearance of the maladjustment syndrome varies: sometimes it may be as short as one or two weeks, sometimes it may be a year. The precipitating factors may be: (1) any illness presenting itself during the struggle for adjustment; (2) any accident, principally if it is a labor accident; (3) bad news from the family: for instance, illness or death of the parents; (4) failure in the job or difficulties with employers or fellow workers; (5) termination of an adaptation achieved with difficulty, e.g., being discharged from a job, necessity for changing living quarters, break up of, or unrequited love affairs.

An amusing observation relevant to the effects of rapid change was made among Hopi Indians in the western United States. A young Hopi, American schooled, may be contrasted with his father. His father believed that when he trod on the tracks of a snake, he would get sore ankles unless he took himself to the medicine man who could prevent this by incantation. This he believed without question, and his visit to the medicine man prevented his ankles from becoming sore. His American-schooled son said he no longer believed in the powers of the medicine man, and considering him a humbug refused to consult him. Nevertheless, he *does* get sore ankles after walking in the tracks of a snake. The implication is that in a rapidly changing society, anxiety-inducing factors outlast anxiety-resolving factors (49-51).

An older and more stable culture is more likely to provide methods for dealing with accumulating tensions, dissatisfactions and conflicts. The development of frustrations and conflicts is minimized in societies where social hierarchies and one's "place in life" are defined, generally known and accepted, and where social stratification is more or less static. The acceptance of what life "hands out" is easier if all those about one are sharing the adverse as well as the satisfying experiences. If, however, it is felt that some groups or individuals are immune to, or unduly protected from the blows of fortune, or if there is a cultural or educational force which suggests that one's lot might be improved, that one is exploited, that the load might be lightened, that those things accepted as inevitable might be avoided if certain steps were taken, there develop conflicts and feelings of frustration, anger, humiliation, and anxiety.

It is of interest that identical protective reaction patterns and their related disease syndromes exhibit themselves in cultural settings exerting almost opposite social pressures. For example, the pressure on the young American male toward emancipation from his parents' authority and toward "standing on his own feet" is in contrast to the Japanese cultural pressure toward parental domination which shapes a young man to assume with filial piety a lifelong obligation and debt to his parents (52). In both cultures some persons, because of highly individual feelings and needs, may not be able to perform in the manner expected of them. The resultant conflict ends in feelings of resentment, guilt, hostility and isolation.

The need to accommodate to a changing world may tax the adaptive capacities of an individual and threaten his security in myriad ways. It is not so much the particular nature of the forces and pressures that threaten, but rather how they are perceived and the amount of conflict directly or indirectly engendered. It is not the specific behavior toward parents, power, possession, sexuality, the hours of work, or even the type of work or the amount of individual freedom of action, but it is the unresolved frustrations and conflict engendered by the culture which become pertinent to the development of stress with its ensuing protective reaction patterns and disease.

Strong support for these inferences was obtained from a careful assessment of the life histories and significant conflicts carried out in a group of 100 non-Communist Chinese students who found themselves literally expatriated in New York during the Revolution in China and in two American groups, one of men and the other of women who included both the most frequently ill and the least frequently ill selected from an industrial population (53, 54). These people were interviewed in the manner developed by Benedict (55, 52) to illuminate the customs and cultural mores of national groups. The subjects were encouraged by "open ended" questions to talk about themselves, their families, their communities, and their attitudes and conflicts.

The interviews were tape recorded and later written out and analysed. This technique which supplemented information from the medical histories and physical examination yielded important information. Although evaluations were made by a number of observers, there was remarkably complete agreement that in all of the cases studied, clusters of illness most often occurred during significantly stress-evoking periods for the individual—when he was striving to adapt to what were for him highly pertinent, conflicting, and often serious threatening demands arising out of his relation to his total environmental constellation, as he perceived it (Fig. 49).

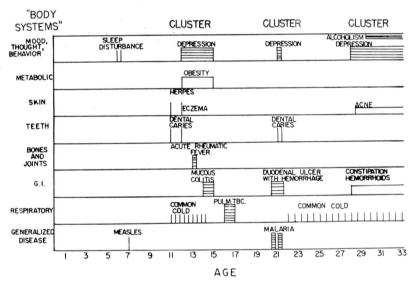

Figure 49. Temporal correlation of illnesses experienced by a Chinese informant over a third of a century.

From the evaluation of the study of the Chinese it can be said that they had shared a life in which they had all been exposed to a rapidly changing culture, repeated disruptions of old social patterns, and many physical dislocations, accompanied by separations from their families and often associated with physical hardships. Again, the healthiest members of this group are people who are able to tolerate with some ease such recurrent disruptions of their life patterns, partly because they regard such changes and disruptions as a normal and expected part of a life pattern, and partly because they are somewhat less involved emotionally in their relationships with other people, and with their goals in life, than is the group in general. Hinkle and Wolff were interested to find that the whole Chinese group had a much greater tolerance for change and disruption than we would expect to see in an equivalent group of Americans and had accepted with relative equanimity dislocations of their life patterns which we would expect to be highly stress-producing for most Americans. This possibly accounted for the fact that the total amount of illness in this group was less than that found in the American working women.

From these general observations upon the three groups, and from the characteristics of the healthiest and unhealthiest members, it appears that the members of these groups who were most healthy were people who were peculiarly well adapted to the particular life situation in which they found themselves, even though there might have been many other life situations to which they could have adapted less well. The opposite was true of those who were most ill. From this, the general inference is made that good health among the informants was the result not of a generally superior adaptive capacity but rather of their having existed in a life situation which satisfied their own peculiar needs and aspirations, however these might differ from those of the population in general. Conversely, Hinkle and Wolff infer that ill health may be evidence of poor adaptive capacity but is not necessarily so; it appears to occur when an individual exists in a life situation which places demands upon him that are excessive in terms of his ability to meet them or which fails to satisfy his own peculiar needs and aspirations.

Many of the least healthy did appear to be people who had been so crippled by their early life experiences or who possessed so many conflicting drives that they could scarcely have adapted to any life situation; but some of the least healthy members of all three groups were persons of outstanding intelligence, superior education, and high standards of conduct, who were resolutely pursuing socially desirable goals in the face of repeated frustrations and overwhelming demands arising out of their life situations.

Some of the healthiest people were those who had spent

their childhood in benign and secure surroundings and who appeared to have learned from their parents consistent patterns of mature behavior in dealing with life crises; and some of these people appeared to have dealt with their needs and the demands of their life situations with outstanding ability. But, there were other healthy people who had encountered a variety of vicissitudes in their childhood environment and who seemed to have no special adaptive capabilities other than those peculiarly suited to the adult environment in which they found themselves; and there were still others who appeared to have maintained their health at the expense of markedly restricting their adult lives, establishing no heterosexual relationships, taking no responsibilities for the welfare of others, and exhibiting an almost pathological opportunism, shallowness of interpersonal relations, and callous indifference to the consequences of their decisions.

In this connection, it is interesting that those who studied surviving American prisoners of war of the Japanese were impressed with the unusually large numbers of individuals who fell at the two extremes of personality integration: on the one end, those who were unusually well adjusted and mature, and on the other, the psychopathic personalities who were able to break the conventional code of moral behavior without suffering guilt and conflict to obtain food and favors from their captors. The highest mortality in the prison camps appeared to occur among those more "normal" individuals who could not adhere to their own standards of conduct, and who, in failing to do so suffered health destroying feelings of anxiety, depression and guilt (56).

All of this we take to confirm our inferences, obtained from the life histories of many individuals, that illness often occurs when an individual perceives his life situation as peculiarly threatening to him, even though this life situation may not appear to be threatening to an outside observer; and that people who maintain good health in a setting of what are "objectively" difficult life situations have within themselves, or can find in their environment, resources with which to balance the difficulties (57, 58).

The study of a community of Italians in the United States, Roseto, Pennsylvania, referred to above, also yielded useful data (41, 42). The town of Roseto had been established in 1882 by

TABLE 1

DEATH RATES PER 100,000 PER YEAR FROM MYOCARDIAL
INFARCTION* BY AGE AND SEX, 1955-1961

Town	Sex	Age Groups					Total
		Under 35	35-44	45-54	55-64	65-Up	
Roseto	M	0	0	144	0	813	91
	F	0	0	0	0	801	66
Nazareth	M	0	0	253	1049	2545	406
	F	0	0	134	234	1309	197
Bangor	M	0	35	305	1082	1866	369
	F	0	58	64	368	1431	244
Stroudsburg	M	42	74	373	910	1980	439
	F	0	0	0	140	695	132
East Stroudsburg	M	0	32	284	705	2344	311
	F	0	0	33	144	689	94

*Proven anatomically and established clinically.

Italian immigrants from a town of the same name in Italy. At first, the Italians were not accepted by their predominantly Anglo-Saxon neighbors and so the community, forced to remain homogeneous and relatively isolated retained much of their Italian peasant way of life. As they perforce became more clannish, they became mutually supporting to the point where there was virtually no crime and no want. They adapted well to the economic circumstances of the United States and some of the families became wealthy. The affluent members, nevertheless, continued to dress and behave in public in the same fashion as their more impecunious neighbors. There was little evidence, therefore, in Roseto of the typical American behavior of "keeping up with the Jones." At the time the study was undertaken, in 1962, the Rosetans had long since been accepted in the larger community of rural Pennsylvania. Indeed, they were often envied for their evident enjoyment of life, their material success and their high community morale. A careful survey of the inhabitants of Roseto revealed, despite their large caloric intake including relatively large quantities of animal fat and their widespread over-weight, an incidence of death from myocardial infarction less than half that of the surrounding community. Together with the lowered death rate was a significantly reduced prevalence of electrocardiographic stigmata of coronary artery disease (118) (Table I).

Through a subsequent study of those born in Roseto who grew up elsewhere in Pennsylvinia or neighboring New York or New Jersey, an attempt was made to sort out genetic, ethnic and cultural factors responsible for the relatively salubrious condition of the people in Roseto. Electrocardiographic evidence of coronary artery disease was found more frequently among relatives who lived elsewhere than among the Rosetans themselves (118, 121). Furthermore, the youngest death from myocardial infarction occurring in Roseto over a span of ten years was in a man age forty-seven, whereas numerous relatives of Rosetans living elsewhere had died in their thirties and forties of myocardial infarction. Thus, although the reasons for the low death rate from myocardial infarction in Roseto are still not fully identified, the social pattern seems to offer more promise of a significant relationship than do genetic or ethnic factors.

Extraordinary opportunities to make ecological studies have been available since the establishment of the State of Israel. Waves of immigrants from seventy-five different nations have converged on Israel, bringing often a relatively homogeous genetic background and centuries of accumulated cultural characteristics, each group contrasting sharply with the other. Already, a wide disparity in the distribution of several diseases has been observed (59). It will now be possible to contrast the state of these groups at the time of immigration to that after aculturation in the Israeli community. Ultimately, the effects of intermarriage and of layering in the new social structure will be accessible to study.

DEPRIVATIONS AND ABUSES

Portentous social challenges grow out of dramatic situations such as wars, civilian catastrophes, explosions, fires, floods and earthquakes. Such events cause major disruptions in the relationships of men and are accompanied not only by epidemics of infectious disease alluded to above but also by such disorders as hypertension, peptic ulcer and endocrine disorders. It is reported that during the three-year long seige of Leningrad during World War II, the prevalence of hypertension rose from 4.1% to 64% in the years 1942-43 (60). Hypertension persisted in most of the victims after the siege was raised and most of them are now dead. An acute catastrophe, the explosion of an ammunition laden tanker in Texas City in 1952 was promptly followed by the appearance of hypertension among a large portion of the citizenry (61).

The incidence of hyperthyroidism in Norway increased one hundred per cent during the first year of World War II when that country was invaded (62). It is also suggestive that other basic endocrine disorders are evident during periods of long-standing chaos (63). Impairment of sexual function with accompanying amenorrhea occurred in nearly all women after internment in the Nazi prison camp of Theresienstadt and in most of the other camps from which reports are available (64).

There is much to be learned from the fact that periods of great duress bring about the decline of some diseases and the increase of others. It seems clear, therefore, that all social challenges do not have equal significance nor do all evoke the same adaptive responses. For example, the successful Dutch merchants mentioned elsewhere (see Chapter IV) who had peptic ulcers before incarceration in German concentration camps lost their stomach lesions under the horrendous conditions that augmented other diseases (64-68). On the other hand, Norwegian and other prisoners of war exposed to extraordinary abuses at the hands of their German or Japanese captors developed a multitude of diseases and disorders reported in order of frequency as edema of malnutrition, serious gastrointestinal disorders, back injuries, head injuries (with loss of consciousness, probably brief) infections of the respiratory tract, infections of the skin, joint pains, loss of weight up to 40 per cent, "encephalitis" and typhus (69).

Among the abuses experienced by jailed prisoners and leading to serious abreactions were long periods of waiting for sentences of death to be executed; being a member of a group the remainder of which had been executed for illegal acts; being members of groups of persons who had to remove unexploded bombs; solitary confinement with periods of great fear during air raids; continued exposure to the gruesome sounds of those being beaten, flogged, guillotined or shot to death. Those who had been in concentration camps described blunting of feelings as a sequel of their suffering, humiliations and deprivations.

Late sequelae of the suffering and misery were major behavior disturbances and even degenerative changes in the brain. Twelve years after the end of World War II many former political prisoners and war veterans had failed to readjust themselves to civil life. Among a group of 100 Norwegians subjected to careful study the breakdowns were noted to have become more frequent as time passed. Those who had been in the concentration camps the longest and had suffered the greatest deprivations and abuses gave evidence of impairment of brain function and structure. Defects were roughly proportional to the duration and intensity of abuse.

Pneumoencephalographic evidence of more or less gross loss of brain substance was found in seventy-five out of eighty-nine subjects so examined. The brain damage that ensued as a sequel of these various noxious factors became manifest regardless of whether or not the prisoner had symptoms of mental impairment during internment or whether he returned to secure personal and social environments thereafter. In many instances, the defects first became evident after the period of internment. The experiences of concentration camps and imprisonment thus appear to have accelerated the aging process.

This study coupled with that made on U.S. prisoners of war lends further support to the view that those who suffer prolonged periods of great duress show great acceleration of the aging process. Loss of brain substance is known to occur with aging. When, as with the chronological age, the duress of daily life is minimal, then relatively few symptoms occur. But should this loss of structure and function occur in younger or middle-aged adults, when the load of daily living is greater, abreactions as in these former prisoners of war may be grave.

There are hints from other sources that years of life can be pressed out of man by catastrophe or prolonged duress. Most physicians have seen sudden and unexplainable death come to those who are overwhelmed or filled with despair. The complex unitary character of mind-body is shown in the evidence that bone pointing, hexing and excommunication of transgressors of tribal mores may remarkably shorten life if not immediately kill a man. Suitable studies still have not been made to explain such deaths. However, it has been shown that wild rats capable of swimming ninety or more hours may, nevertheless, die in a few minutes when they have been terrified before being plunged into water. Careful study of the hearts of these creatures revealed that death resulted from a depressive reaction of the nervous system which gradually slowed and ultimately arrested the heart's beat. But, when the rat was lifted from the water shortly before the heart stopped, it promptly recovered and could withstand subsequent immersions better than an average rat (70).

The oxygen conserving reflex described in Chapter III, page 74, may be pertinent to the mechanism of death observed in the rats. It is elicited most characteristically by immersion of the face in water. Sudden bradycardia is a striking feature of the reflex. Like other reaction patterns designed to deal with a particular kind of danger, the oxygen conserving reflex may be elicited under circumstances perhaps grave, but which do not necessarily imply the likelihood of a shortage of oxygen. It may be that instances of sudden death in man can be attributed to such a reflex slowing of the heart gone beyond the limits of survival (71, 72).

Early information from Japan, as yet statistically unsupported, indicates that those who experienced the catastrophe of the atom bomb at Hiroshima but who themselves suffered no burns or direct effects of irradiation have had a shorter life span that other Japanese. Death has resulted from the usual and varied terminal illnesses. It is as though they had grown twenty years older than their actual age (73).

Though definite support for this early impression awaits further statistical analysis, we do have precise information from our own records of World War II and the Korean action concerning the effect on life span and health of prolonged adverse and seriously threatening life experience (56). Of approximately 7,000 United States prisoners of war captured by the North Koreans, about one-third died. Medical observers reported that the cause of death in many instances was ill-defined and was referred to by the prisoners as "give up-itis." Death seemed to be the end result of depletion, starvation, cold, dysentery, pneumonia, exhaustion, serious demoralization, humiliation, despair, and deprivation of human support and affection. The prisoner simply became apathetic, listless, neither ate nor drank, helped himself in no way, stared into space, and finally died.

A recently completed study of the effects of imprisonment on Americans during World War II (74) furnishes revealing information about approximately 94,000 United States prisoners of war who were taken in Europe. These men were imprisoned for about ten months. Less than one per cent of them died before liberation. In contrast, in the Pacific theatre, about 25,000 Americans became prisoners of war. They remained in prison four times as long as those captured in Europe and suffered far more threats, abuse, and humiliation. Their demoralization was often extreme. More than one-third of them died in prison.

Six years after liberation, the fate of those that survived the Japanese prison experience was investigated. In the first place, the total number of deaths in the group during these six years was more than twice the expected incidence for a similar group of persons not so exposed and three times as great as in the group of United States prisoners of war in Europe. Moreover, the causes of death included many diseases not directly related to confinement or starvation: twice the expected number of heart disease, more than twice the expected number of cancer, and more than four times the expected number of diseases of the gastro-intestinal tract. Twice the number died from suicide—and most striking of all, three times the expected number died as a result of accidents. Nine times the expected number died of pulmonary tuberculosis (74).

What was the incidence of illness during the six years after their liberation? It was found that the admission rate to veterans' hospitals among former prisoners of war of the Japanese was closely related to the amount of stress endured during imprisonment. Those who had experienced less duress had admission rates only slightly higher than the European prisoners of war. But, those who had suffered greatly had far the greatest number of admissions—amounting to seven times as many as did those who had not been prisoners—and "very poor health" interfered with work in one half. Those who were in "very poor health" had many different diseases, among them many that did not appear to be immediately related to incarceration, such as hernia, deafness, and diseases of bones, muscles, and heart. There were ten times as many impairments as among the European prisoners of war.

STRESS-PRODUCING FACTORS IN
THE AMERICAN CULTURE

Important as are the upheavals of rapid social change and the cruel circumstances imposed on man by his fellows, the ordinary vicissitudes of daily life offer their share of challenge as has been pointed out. It may indeed be stated that man is always under stress of one sort or another. Modern man feels himself under more stress than his progenitors. At any rate, he manifests his state conspicuously and complains about it freely. We may ask: what brings about such stress in our culture at this time? The situation in the U.S.A. may be selected for focus. Sociologists have suggested that while our society is passing through a phase of rapidly changing norms* and mores**, the individual members are made anxious by the newer cultural pressures added to displacement of the older and without the benefit of the latter's anxiety-resolving devices. Thus as in the case of the Hopi Indian, the participant proceeds without confidence, having lost faith in the old guides. There is no precedent for the changing protocols, his parents, teachers and elders no longer speak with authority, and he is too often left to his own devices. He mistrusts his habits and intuitions, and social experience no longer leads to a "common sense" of values.

Along with this loss of anchorage, comes pressure to develop independence, show initiative and shape one's world. The Promethean attitude is emphasized: "steps must be taken," "something must be done about it," obstacles must be overcome, the environment changed, and the pressure removed by a plan, a procedure, a committee, an organization. Also, emphasis is on modification of the "outside" world; cooling the environment when it is hot, warming it when cold, carrying water to where there is none, bearing minerals from arid areas to grow fruit in fertile zones, moving mountains, tapping the earth's energy. In short, "to bend the external world of men and things according to his predilections" (75). In such a culture, to accept deprivations, discomforts, inconveniences, compromises, and so to change one's attitudes and appetites as to develop acceptance, endurance and tolerance, is considered inappropriate, lacking in initiative and unbecoming in a man. In short, internal rearrangement or changing in attitude runs counter to an important cultural direction.

To the queries, "how much do I have to put up with?" "am I a sucker to take this?" the culture answers that a man must take action and change his environment. Industrialization (76)

---

*Norms—that which "ought" or "should" be done or that which one is expected to do.

**Mores—customs, ways of doing.

with its attendant migrations and movements to and among cities
becomes an aspect of this way of life and, as well, gives scope for
its development (77-84). Family disorganization (85-91), altered
relations between the sexes, lack of conviction of "roots," of
"belonging," and decline in "purpose" are further and untoward
expressions of the present day cultural patterns (92-96). It is
indeed striking that the substantial rewards achieved in this new
society, even though the individuals proclaim "happiness," do not
appear to compensate at deep biological and spiritual levels for
the losses. The titillations, bounties, "conveniences," "freedoms,"
and excitements seem superficial in their constructive effects as
compared with the potential destructiveness of rapid cultural
change. Hence, the paradox of "sick" though ostensibly "improved" man.

With the lusty clamor for freedom all over the world, with
telephone communication between the Antipodes, with common
markets erasing boundaries and with jet propelled travel within
hours to everywhere it is indeed difficult to be a citizen wherever
the old codes are being jettisoned. Rapid social change is a
universal phenomenon in this aging twentieth century.

MAN-WOMAN RELATIONSHIPS AND THE FAMILY

One of the most basic changes which has characterized the
development of modern society is a disruption of the family and
a reorientation of the Man-Woman relationship. For centuries,
whatever occupation was assumed by the male in a given society
has been accorded preeminence and prestige in the eyes of his
spouse. Before our day, a woman, within the walls of her home
and in relation to the procreative family, has conceded the "number one" position to her mate, whether or not she may have
outstripped her marital partner in any life activity, and regardless of her relative capacity in competition with other men and
women and of her importance in the community outside of the
home. The man, on the other hand, historically has been willing
to assume the "number one" role. Nowadays, domestic state itself
is threatened and in danger of collapse because no longer are such
concessions made, so that the man and his role are accepted as
dominant.

Although there are extremes in the completeness with which these generalizations are exhibited in any one culture, it is likely if a sufficiently large number and variety of cultures were studied and appraised, that the above principles would prevail. In any event, our own rapidly changing culture exhibits uncertainty concerning these relationships and consequent instability in family life (87-89).

Great additional burdens are thrown upon the marital partner and the physician since they are among the few surviving sources of security in a rapidly changing culture. The physician must carry not only the load assumed by his professional fore-bears, but also the greatly added load created by default of other anxiety-resolving agents in society. The church, the school, the recreation center, the teacher, the police, the social worker, the clergy cannot replace the security engendered by stable family life (97-99). The world awaits with justified curiosity the ultimate outcome of the disruption of the centuries-old family system in Red China.

PEPTIC ULCERATION AND CHANGE

The reversed sex incidence of peptic ulcers with perforations is a dramatic exhibition of the repercussions of a changing social order on the relations of the sexes and the subsequent effects on health. Jennings (100) investigated the age, incidence, and sex distribution of a large series of patients with peptic ulcers outside the United States in the last 150 years. The lesions were not visualized in all individuals, but the evidence for diagnosis seemed convincing. Between 1850 and 1900, of every six patients with peptic ulcers perforated into the peritoneal cavity, four were women and two were men. Since 1920, of every ten perforations, one has occurred in an elderly woman and nine have occurred in men, mostly in the middle years or younger.

A review (101) of the incidence of perforated ulcer at the New York Hospital from 1880 to 1900 revealed that women had perforated ulcer about as commonly as men, i.e., seven men to six women. All perforations in these patients were visualized either at operation or autopsy (all autopsies from 1880 to 1891). Beginning in the period of 1901 through 1906 the ratio of males

to females began to increase. The following figures were found
for the years 1901-1939:

		Males	Females	Ratio
1901 - 1906	(5 years)	10	4	2.5:1 - 2.5
1907 - 1914	(7 years)	55	9	6:1 - 6.0
1915 - 1930	(15 years)	260	16	16:1 - 16.0
1932 through 1939	(8 years)	36	3	12:1 - 12.0

Thus, perforations of ulcers in young women occurred frequently in the nineteenth century and diminished relatively at
the beginning of the twentieth century. Statistics revealing
similar ratios have been compiled by Alsted (102) and, according
to Jennings, increase in the ratio of males to females has taken
place in Germany, France, Scandinavia and the English-speaking
countries (100). Uncomplicated ulcers probably fall into the
same category as perforated ulcers.

Whether or not there has been an absolute increase in peptic
ulcer in relation to the total population is irrelevant to the fact
that during the last half century peptic ulcer has become principally a male disorder.

Can this be understood in terms of a changed relationship
between the sexes? There is much to suggest that it can. Interpersonal and social pressures that evoke particular kinds of
attitudes and reactions have been shown elsewhere in this essay
to be extremely pertinent to the production and exacerbation of
peptic ulceration. The adjustments imposed by decline in religious faith, by reduction of the family to the procreative unit
and the deterioration of the larger family relations (loss of
intimate contact with cousins, uncles, and aunts in the community) ; by the rise of urbanization with the loss of neighbor-
liness in the large, impersonal and shifting residential zones
about industries, all throw more and more of a burden upon the
residual institutions that engender security. Of outstanding
significance is the change, during this period, of women's attitude
toward men. As indicated above, entirely unpremeditated changes
in our social pattern have been precipitated by urbanization
and its effects on the relations within the family. The ensuing
changes in women's social status have resulted (for the most part

fortunately) in a challenge to the male position of "dominance" which was taken for granted in the nineteenth century.

The prestige for women was gained mainly through marriage. Indeed, in the nineteenth century if a woman were not married in her early twenties her position was exceedingly difficult. Her period of maximum striving and competitive effort toward marriage was between seventeen and twenty-seven. If by this time she had not married, she became a subservient figure in some relative's home. The cultural pattern for female behavior fostered stress by strictly limiting a woman's goals and denying her overt expression of her competitive effort.

After marriage, the relationship between a man and a woman was well defined. A man was freely conceded the "number one" position in his home and was expected to be "master" in his household, yet within this pattern of male dominance men were permitted considerable emotional dependence upon their women. Under cover of his "dominant" position a man could give free expression to his emotional need. His idiosyncrasies were indulged and his peccadilloes tolerated.

With the change in cultural values, however, a man's position in the family became less clear. A woman might be the most important financial contributor to the home, in which case she often unwittingly created in her partner a conviction of inadequacy. If she failed in an occupational venture, she was justified by society in retiring and being provided for by her husband. Such provision for a man has no social approval. If a man fails to be a "good provider," he may be denied the feeling of security which his wife's emotional support could give him. Indeed, a wife's humiliation of her husband under circumstances of his failure to "provide" is endorsed by cultural sanctions. Thus, while society's requirements of the male are essentially as stringent as before, the emotional support accorded him in return has become less. The changes in women affect not only their husbands, but also their children, especially their sons, because there has been created in the home a background of challenge, irresponsibility and unpredictability.

In brief, with the social changes that occurred during the early part of the present century men have been confronted with decreasing opportunities for emotional support, yet their responsibilities have remained and the threats to their self-esteem have increased. The shift of primary incidence in peptic ulceration from female to male may be related to these changes.

Since mid-century, there is some evidence that the relative prevalence of duodenal ulcer among women may have increased reducing the degree of the male-female discrepancy. During the years 1957 to 1962, the male-female ratio of peptic ulcer diagnosed at New York Hospital was approximately three to one. Much more extensive data are available from the National Health survey of 235,000 persons in 73,000 household interviews covering the period July 1, 1957 through June 1959. The prevalence of peptic ulcer in the various age groups is shown in Table 2. Here again, the ratio of males to females was approximately three to one (103). This recent change in the relative numbers of peptic ulcers among men and women suggests the inference that women's full access to her "rights" and increasing opportunities to compete in a world of affairs may carry identical emotional pitfalls for her as for the man whose bodily and emotional comforts she has neglected in order to have her own career. (Table II)

The nature of the relationship between man and wife determines in large part the quality of the social milieu of the child. Freud focused attention on the deep and lasting effects of the conflicts and anxieties created by parental figures in their offspring. It then follows that the anxieties and conflicts engendered in the parents by cultural pressures (104, 90, 105) through which they have suffered frustration and rejection, are projected on their children. The parents' hostilities, their subsequent limited capacity to give and accept love are features of their own insecurity, promptly reflecting themselves in the family relationships, Also, children readily perceive when, for the parents, the "breath of life" is going out of a deteriorating family relationship concerning which the parents yet remain irresolute. The phenomenon of the revolt of the children and their rejection of parents then becomes as conspicuous as parents vascillation in

TABLE 2
PREVALENCE PER 1,000 OF PEPTIC ULCER

Age	Male	Female	Ratio Males to Females
All ages	21.4	7.7	2.8
0 - 24	—	—	—
25 - 34	29.3	7.0	4.2
35 - 44	42.5	13.9	3.1
45 - 54	40.5	17.5	2.3
55 - 64	39.0	14.2	2.7
65+	33.0	13.3	2.5

rejecting the whole responsibility of family life, and children in particular. This sad state of affairs threatens the security, and indeed the health, of all individuals concerned.

Intensive study of an American community (104) allows us to examine the cultural factors more closely. Half consciously and unconsciously motivated behavior not only stems from basic strivings having to do with sex appetites and needs, and unrecognized hostilities in relation to punitive parents, but also with the frustrations from social striving experienced by the members of ostensibly "mobile"* society. In the U.S.A., for example, where "getting ahead" is so important, frustrations, anxieties and resentments are often unconsciously experienced by the members of this highly stratified society which has developed and made a myth of our being a "one-class, middle-class" nation (104, 106, 107). Indeed, it is a common belief held by Americans that at least 80 per cent are in the "middle class." Yet, as indicated by Warner in his "Yankee City" studies (104), more than one half of a typical community has been classified as "lower."

Least conflict, striving and competitiveness are found in the two social extremes, the highest and the lowest groups, since in both mere maintenance of status is usually considered sufficient (54). But, in the intermediate classes, and especially as regards movement from lower into middle, and upward movement within the middle class, striving and competitiveness are a dominant aspect of day to day living. It involves "improvement" in education, in occupation, in money income, in residence, and in the assumption of new behavioral patterns.

Serious problems for the children may evolve not only from the disrupted household but in the case of even the most devoted family, the pressures of society for "success" in the children of "successful" parents may create insurmountable difficulties for the children. In this connection also, the ambitions of parents for their children, and the pressures often unwittingly put upon them to match or even exceed the upward progress of a parent may force the offspring into an impossible dilemma. Individual

---
*"Mobile"—ease of movement from one social stratum to another.

proclivities, capabilities and appetites no longer have free play. Achievement becomes elusive because of conflicting and oftimes unattainable goals. In such a soil, bitter and paralyzing frustration with resentment and even hatred for the parents, may flourish.

The many and various ethnic groups introduced into the U.S.A. in the late nineteenth and early twentieth centuries have had the double task of becoming incorporated into a new and different culture, which is in itself rapidly changing, and then moving up from stratum to stratum in that culture. Reference points for them have thus become especially ill defined.

Striking though these factors be in the U.S.A. where intensive sociological study is continually illuminating them, it is likely that increasing industrialization and urbanization of European countries have created similar social reorganization, strivings, competitiveness and conflicts. Not only common to all contemporary Western culture but also in emerging nations all around the world are varying degrees of industrialization, urbanization (79-81, 108, 109), centralization through organization, social mobility, and changing values. One may profitably ask whether man has ever been called upon to change his ways on so large a scale and so rapidly. Intimately related to these changes and perhaps most significant to the health of man are the disorganization and attempts at reorganization of family life as well as more mundane changes in social arrangements as already referred to in the work of Rahe and Holmes (117).

Studies already made of the relevance of adaptive and protective patterns to health and disease warrant the following inferences. Man's relation to his social environment has a major influence upon his health. His attempts to adapt to life situations which do not fulfill his needs, which frustrate his aspirations, or which place heavy and conflicting demands upon him are very often associated with an increased susceptibility to all forms of illness, regardless of nature or etiology, and they may be associated with the development of life-endangering or permanently crippling pathological processes. In the population in general, those who are having difficulty in adapting to challenging life situations are those who exhibit a major proportion of the illnesses occurring in the adult population. The further investigation of how man's relation to his social environment affects his health should be among the foremost concerns of those in the field of medicine and public health.

BIBLIOGRAPHY

1. HINKLE, L. E., and WOLFF, H. G.: Communist interrogation and indoctrination of "enemies of the state." Analysis of methods used by the Communist State Police (A special report). *Arch. Neurol. Psychiat.*, 76:115-174, 1956.

2. HINKLE, L. E., and WOLFF, H. G.: The nature of man's adaptation to his total environment and the relation of this to illness. *Arch. Intern. Med.*, 99:442-460, 1957.

3. SCHOTTSTAEDT, W. W., PINSKY, R. H., MACKLER, D., and WOLF, S.: Sociologic, psychologic and metabolic observations of patients in the community of a metabolic ward. *Amer. J. Med.*, 25:248, 1958.

4. SCHOTTSTAEDT, W. W., PINSKY, R. H., MACKLER, D., and WOLF, S.: Prestige and social interaction on a metabolic ward. *Psychosom. Med.*, 21:131, 1959.

5. SCHOTTSTAEDT, W. W., JACKMAN, N. R., McPHAIL, C. S., and WOLF, S.: Social interaction on a metabolic ward; the relation of problems of status to chemical balance. *J. Psychosom. Res.*, 7:83-95, 1963.

6. SCHOTTSTAEDT, W. W., and WOLF, S.: The evaluation of psychologic factors in illness. *Med. Clin. N. Amer.*, 46:859-864, 1962.

7. WOLF, STEWART: The implications of social sciences for the future of medicine. In: *Medical Education and Medical Care: Interactions and Prospects*, Chap. 2. Report of 8th Teaching Institute, Assn. of Am. Med. Colleges, Evanston, 1961.

8. BERNARD, CLAUDE: *Leçons sur les Propriétés Physiologiques et les Altérations Pathologiques des Liquides de l'Organisme*. Paris, Bailleurs, 1859.

9. SECHENOV, IVAN: *Reflexes of the Brain* (Moscow, 1873) Reprinted by Idz—Vo Academy of Medicine, USSR, 1952.

10. HIPPOCRATES: *Works of Hippocrates. Medical Classics*. New York, 1938, Vol. 3, pp. 299-381.

11. ARMSTRONG, C., and WOOLEY, J. G.: Studies of newly discovered virus which causes lymphocytic choriomeningitis in experimental animals. *Pub. Health Report, 50*:537-541, 1935.

12. TRAUB, E.: Filterable virus recovered from white mice. *Science, 81*:298-299, 1935.

13. ANDREWES, C. H., and GLOVER, R. E.: Grey lung virus: Agent pathogenic for mice and other rodents. *Brit. J. Exp. Path., 26*:379-387, 1945.

14. THOMAS, L., and KOLK, E. M.: Activation of latent mouse pneumonitis virus by human serum. *Proc. Soc. Exp. Biol. Med., 55*:1-4, 1944.

15. NIGG, C., and EATON, M. D.: Isolation from normal mice of pneumotropic virus which forms elementary bodies. *J. Exp. Med., 79*:497-510, 1944.

16. MEYER, K. F.: The ecology of psittacosis and ornithosis. *Medicine, 21*:175, 1942.

17. SHOPE, R. E.: Swine lungworm as reservoir and intermediate host for swine influenza virus; demonstration of masked swine influenza virus in lungworm larvae and swine under natural conditions. *J. Exp. Med., 77*:127-138, 1943.

18. KOPROWSKI, HILARY: Latent or dormant viral infections. *Ann. N.Y. Acad. Sci., 54*:963-976, 1952.

19. BLANK, H., and BRODY, M. W.: Recurrent herpes simplex. A psychiatric and laboratory study. *Psychosom. Med., 12*:254, 1950.

20. HEILIG, R., and HOFF, H.: Ueber psychogenen Entstehung des Herpes Labialis. *Med. Klin., 24*:1472, 1928.

21. SCHNECK, J. M.: The psychological components in a case of Herpes Simplex. *Psychosom. Med., 9*:62, 1947.

22. SCHWARTZMAN, G., and ARONSON, S. A.: Studies on the extraneural phase of experimental poliomyelitis. Program, American Academy of Neurology, 5th Annual Meeting, April 9-11, 1953. Chicago, Illinois.

23. DUBOS, RENE: *Mirage of Health; Utopias, Progress and Biological Change.* New York, Harper, 1959.

24. DUBOS, RENE: *The Germ Theory Revisited.* Lecture delivered at Cornell University Medical College, New York, March 18, 1953. *Cornell Special Lecture Series.*

25. SIGERIST, HENRY E.: *Man and Medicine.* Trans. by Margaret Galt Boise. New York, Norton, 1932, p. 180.

26. DuBos, Rene: Personal communication to H. G. Wolff, 1951.
27. McDougal, J. B.: *Tuberculosis—A Global Study in Social Pathology*. Baltimore, Williams and Wilkins, 1949.
28. Krause, Allen K.: Factors in the pathogenesis of tuberculosis. *Amer. Rev. Tuberc., 18*:208, 1928.
29. Krause, Allen K.: Tuberculosis and public health. *Amer. Rev. Tuberc., 18*:271, 1928.
30. DuBos, R. J.: Biological and social aspects of tuberculosis. *Bull. N.Y. Acad. Med., 27*:351, 1951.
31. DuBos, R. J.: The tubercle bacillus and tuberculosis. *Amer. Sci., 37*:353, 1949.
32. Wolf, George: Tuberculosis mortality and industrialization. *Amer. Rev. Tuberc., 42*:1, 1940.
33. Adams, W. F.: *Ireland and Irish Emigration to the New World.* New Haven, Yale, 1932.
34. Drolet, G. J.: Epidemiology of tuberculosis. In: *Clinical Tuberculosis*, B. Goldberg, Ed. Philadelphia, Davis, 1946.
35. Moorman, Lewis J.: Tuberculosis on the Navaho Reservation. *Amer. Rev. Tuberc., 61*:586, 1950.
36. Holmes, T. H., Hawkins, N. G., Bowerman, C. E., Clarke, E. R., and Joffe, J. R.: Psychosocial and psychophysiologic studies of tuberculosis. *Psychosom. Med., 19*:134, 1957.
37. Sartwell, P. E., and Smith, W. M.: Epidemiological notes on meningococcal meningitis in the army. *Amer. J. Public Health, 34*:40-49, 1944.
38. Bakke, J. L., and Wolff, H. G.: Life situations and serum antibody titers. *Psychosom. Med., 10*:327, 1948.
39. DuBos, Rene: Studies on the mechanism of a specific bacterial enzyme which decomposes the capsular polysaccharide of Type III pneumococcus. *J. Exp. Med., 62*:259, 1935.
40. Christenson, W. N., and Hinkle, L. E., Jr.: Differences in illness and prognostic signs in two groups of young men. Abstract, American Federation of Clinical Research, April 30, 1960.
41. Hampton, J., Stout, C., Brandt, E., and Wolf, S.: Prevalence of myocardial infarction and related diseases in an Italian-American community. Abstract *J. Lab. Clin. Med., 64*:866, 1964.
42. Stout, Clarke, Morrow, Jerry, Brandt, E. N., and Wolf, S.: Unusually low incidence of death from myocardial infarction. Study of an Italian-American community in Pennsylvania. *J.A.M.A., 188*:845-849, 1964.

43. CANNON, W. B.: Voodoo death. *Amer. Anthrop., 44*:169, 1942.
44. WOLF, S., BIRD, R. M., and SMITH, JAMES J.: Personal observations during World War II on New Guinea.
45. SAINSBURY, PETER: *Suicide in London* (Maudsley Monograph, No. 1) New York, Basic Books, 1956.
46. GOODELL, H.: Unpublished studies on suicide rates in the U.S.A.
47. WOLFF, H. G.: Changes in vulnerability of tissue: An aspect of man's response to threat. The National Institute of Health, Annual Lectures, 1953, pp. 38-71. U.S. Dept. of Health, Education and Welfare, Publication #388.
48. SEGUIN, C. ALBERTO: Migration and psychosomatic disadaptation. *J. Psychosom. Med., 18*:404-409, 1956.
49. SIMMONS, L. W.: The relation between the decline of anxiety-inducing and anxiety-resolving factors in a deteriorating culture and its relevance to bodily disease. *Proc. Ass. Res. Nerv. Ment. Dis., 29*:127, 1950.
50. SIMMONS, L. W.: *Sun Chief.* 2nd Ed., New Haven, Yale, 1947.
51. SIMMONS, L. W., and WOLFF, H. G.: *Social Science in Medicine.* New York, Russell Sage Foundation, 1954.
52. BENEDICT, RUTH: *The Chrysanthemum and the Sword: Patterns of Japanese Culture.* Boston, Houghton, 1946.
53. HINKLE, L. E., JR., GITTINGER, J., GOLDBERGER, L., OSTFELD, A., METRAUX, R., RICHTER, P., and WOLFF, H. G.: Studies in human ecology: Factors governing the adaptation of Chinese unable to return to China. In: *Experimental Psychopathology.* New York, Gune and Stratton, 1957, Chap. II, pp. 170-186.
54. HINKLE, L. E., JR., and WOLFF, H. G.: Health and social environment: Experimental investigations. In: *Explorations in Social Psychiatry.* Leighton, Clausen and Wilson, Eds. New York, Basic Books, 1957.
55. BENEDICT, RUTH: *Patterns of Culture* (with a new preface by Margaret Mead). Boston, Houghton, 1959 (1934).
56. WOLF, S. and RIPLEY, H. S.: Reactions among Allied prisoners of war subjected to three years of imprisonment and torture by the Japanese. *Am. J. Psych., 104*:180, 1947.
57. WOLFF, H. G.: What hope does for man. Science and Humanity Section. Saturday Rev., pp. 42-45, 1956 (Also reprinted and distributed by N. Y. State Committee on TB and P.H. and N. Y. State Heart Assn., Inc.) Also see: Has disease meaning? *Soc. N. Y. Hosp. Rec.,* May 8, 1956, pp. 10-17.

58. WOLFF, H. G.: Stressors as a cause of disease in man. Chapt. 2, Disorganization of behavior in man, pp. 17-31, in: *Stress and Psychiatric Disorder*, J. M. Tanner, Ed. Oxford, Blackwell, 1960.

59. GROEN, J. J., and LIEBER, E.: Socio-medical aspects of bronchial asthma in Israel. *Israel Med. J., 19*:121-36, 1960.

60. VALDMAN, CHERNORUTSKII, LANG-BELONOGOVA: Quoted by Hoffmann, B.: Blood pressure and subarctic climate in the Soviet Union (Survey of the Russian Literature and Investigations on Delayed Repatriots). (English transl. by E. A. White Res. Assoc., I.C.R.S., Fordham Univ., New York.) Publ., Prof. Dr. Med., Max Brandt, East Europe Hist. of Berlin Free Univ., Medical Series 16, 1958.

61. RUSKIN, A. BERNARD, O. W., and SCHAFFER, R. L.: Blast hypertension. Elevated arterial pressure in the victims of the Texas city disaster. *Amer. J. Med., 4*:288, 1948.

62. GREILAND, R.: Thyrotoxicosis at Ulleval Hospital in the years 1934-1944, with a special view to frequency of the disease. *Act. Med. Scand., 125*:108, 1946.

63. SELYE, H.: *Textbook of Endocrinology*, Ed. II. Montreal, Acta Endocrinologica, Inc., 1950.

64. COHEN, E. A.: *Human Behavior in the Concentration Camp*. London, Jonathan Cape, 1954.

65. GROEN, J., et al.: *Psychosomatic Research*. London, Pergamon Press, 1964.

66. GROEN, J. J.: Personal communication.

67. GROEN, J. J.: *Psychopathogenese van Ulcus Ventriculi et Duodeni*. Amsterdam, Scheltema and Holkema, 1947.

68. GROEN, J. J.: Personal communication.

69. KRAL, V. A.: Psychiatric observations under severe chronic stress. *Amer. J. Psychiat., 108*:135, 1951.

70. RICHTER, CURT P.: On the phenomenon of sudden death in animals and man. *Psychosom. Med., 19*:191-198, 1957.

71. WOLF, S.: The bradycardia of the dive reflex—A possible mechanism of sudden death. *Trans. Amer. Clin. Climat. Ass., 76*: 192, 1964.

72. WOLF, S., SCHNEIDER, ROBERT A., and GROOVER, M. E., JR.: Further studies on the circulatory and metabolic alterations of the oxygen-conserving (diving) reflex in man. *Trans. Ass. Amer. Physicians, 78*:242, 1965.

73. SHIRABE, R.: Medical survey of atomic bomb casualties, p. 1-27, Oak Ridge National Laboratory. Atomic Energy Commission, April, 1954.

74. COHEN, BERNARD M., and COOPER, MAURICE Z.: A follow-up study of World War II Prisoners of War. VA Medical Monograph, VA Administration and National Research Council, Committee on Veterans Medical Problems, Washington, 1954.

75. HSU, F. L. K.: *The Chinese Hawaii.* Trans. by *New York Acad. Sci., 13*:243, 1951.

76. CARSKADON, THOMAS R., and MODLEY, RUDOLPH: *U.S.A. Measure of a Nation.* New York, MacMillan, 1949.

77. NATIONAL RESOURCES PLANNING BOARD: *Problems of a Changing Population,* Washington, D. C., 1938.

78. OGBURN, W. F., and NIMKOFF, M. F.: *Sociology.* New York, Houghton, 1950.

79. GIST, N. P., and HALBERT, L. A.: *Urban Society,* New York, Crowell, 1933, 1940 and 1948.

80. MUMFORD, LEWIS: *The Culture of Cities.* New York, Harcourt, 1938.

81. JACOBS, JANE: *Death and Life of Great American Cities.* New York, Random, 1961.

82. VANCE, RUPERT B.: *Research Memorandum on Population Redistribution within the United States.* Research Council Bulletin 42, New York, 1938.

83. LANDIS, PAUL H.: *Population Problems, A Cultural Interpretation.* New York, American Book, 1943.

84. DAVIS, KINGSLEY: *Human Society.* New York, MacMillan, 1949.

85. LYND, R. S. and LYND, HELEN M.: *Middletown (1929) and Middletown in Transition (1937).* New York, Harcourt.

86. LUMPKIN, KATHERINE P.: *The Family, A Study in Member Roles.* Chapel Hill, Univ. N. Carolina Press, 1933.

87. TRUXAL, ANDREW G., and MERRILL, FRANCIS E.: *The Family in American Culture.* New York, Prentice-Hall, 1947.

88. MOWRER, E. R.: *Family Disorganization.* Chicago, Univ. Chicago Press, 1927.

89. HAMILTON, G. V.: *Research in Marriage.* New York, Albert and Charles Boni, 1929.

90. BOSSARD, JAMES H.: *The Sociology of Child Development.* New York, Harper, 1950.

91. BERLE, BEATRICE B.: *80 Porto Rican Families in New York City; Health and Disease Studied in Context.* New York, Columbia Univ. Press, 1958.

92. COOLEY, CHARLES H.: *Social Organization.* New York, Scribner, 1909.

93. CURTI, M., SHRYOCK, R. H., COCHRAN, T. C., and HARRINGTON, F. H.: *An American History.* Vol. 2. New York, Harper, 1950.

94. GROETHUYSEN, B.: Secularism. *Encyclopedia of the Social Sciences.* Vol. 13, New York, MacMillan, 1937.

95. PLANT, JAMES S.: *Personality and the Culture Pattern.* New York, Commonwealth Fund, 1937.

96. GLAZER, NATHAN, and MOYNIHAN, DANIEL PATRICK: *Beyond the Melting Pot.* Cambridge, Massachusetts Institute of Technology Press, 1963.

97. MEAD, MARGARET: *Male and Female. A Study of the Sexes in a Changing World.* New York, Morrow, 1949.

98. MEAD, MARGARET: *Sex and Temperament in Three Primitive Societies.* New York, Morrow, 1935.

99. MEAD, MARGARET: *Family.* New York, MacMillan, 1965.

100. JENNINGS, D.: Perforated peptic ulcer. Changes in age-incidence and sex distribution in the last 150 years. *Lancet, 1*:395, 1940.

101. MITTELMANN, B., and WOLFF, H. G.: Emotions and gastroduodenal function: Experimental studies on patients with gastritis, duodenitis and peptic ulcer. *Psychosom. Med., 4*:5-61, 1942.

102. ALSTED, G.: *Studies on the Changing Incidence of peptic ulcer of the stomach and duodenum.* Humphrey Milford, London, Oxford, 1939.

103. KOVAR, MARY GRACE: Peptic ulcers reported in interviews, June, 1957-June, 1959 Series B., No. 17, Health Statistics, U.S. National Health Survey, U.S. Dept. of Health, Education and Welfare, Public Health Service, Washington, D.C., June, 1960.

104. WARNER, W. L., and LUNT, P. S.: *The Social Life of a Modern Community* (Yankee City Series, Vol. 1) New Haven, Yale, 1947.

105. HARING, DOUGLAS G., Ed.: *Personal Character and Cultural Milieu.* Syracuse, Syracuse Univ. Press, 1949.

106. CENTERS, RICHARD: The American class structure: A psychological analysis. In: *Readings in Social Psychology.* T. M. Newcomb, and E. L. Hartley, Eds. New York, Holt, 1947.

107. *The People of the U.S.A.—A Self Portrait.* Fortune Magazine. February, 1940, pp. 14, 28.
108. National Resources Committee: *Our Cities: Their Role in the National Economy.* Washington, D. C., June, 1937.
109. MUNRO, WILLIAM B.: *City.* In: *Encyclopedia of the Social Sciences.* Vol. 3, New York, MacMillan, 1930.
110. WOLFF, H. G.: Dormant human potential. *Arch. Neurol., 6*:261-263, 1962.
111. WOLF, S.: A new view of disease. *Trans. Amer. Clin. Climat. Ass., 74*:168-175, 1963. *J. Amer. Med. Ass., 184(2)*:129, 1963.
112. WOLFF, H. G.: The mind-body relationship. In: *An Outline of Man's Knowledge.* New York, Doubleday, 1960, Chap. 2, pp. 43-72.
113. WOLF, S.: Ecology and the spirit of man. In: *Psychiatry in Medicine.* Norman Q. Brill, Ed. Los Angeles, Univ. Calif. Press, 1962, Chap. 5.
114. BYKOV, K. M.: The cerebral cortex and the internal organs. W. Horsley Gantt, Trans and Ed. New York, Chemical Publishing, (Reviewed by H. G. Wolff, *J. Psychosom. Res., 4*:56, 1959).
115. WOLF, S.: Human values. *J.A.M.A., 180*:56, 1962.
116. WOLF, S.: The expectations of society. *J. Med. Educ., 40(1)*:3, 1965.
117. RAHE, R. H., MEYER, M., SMITH, M., KJAER, G. and HOLMES, T. H.: Social stress and illness onset. *J. Psychosom. Res., 8*:35, 1965.
118. BRANDT, E. N., STOUT, CLARKE, HAMPTON, JAMES W., LYNN, THOMAS N. and WOLF, S.: Coronary heart disease among Italians and non-Italians in Roseto, Pennsylvania, and in nearby communities. Chapter 28 in: *Prevention of Ischemic Heart Disease,* Wilhelm Raab, Ed. Springfield, Ill., Thomas, 1966.
119. BRUHN, J., CHANDLER, B., MILLER, C. and LYNN, T.: Social aspects of coronary heart disease in two adjacent, ethnically different communities. *Amer. J. Public Health, 56*:1493, 1966.
120. BRUHN, JOHN: An epidemiological study of myocardial infarctions in an Italian-American community. *J. Chronic Dis., 18*:353, 1965.
121. LYNN, T., DUNCAN, R., NAUGHTON, J., WULFF, J., BRANDT, E. and WOLF, S.: Prevalence of Evidence of Prior Myocardial Infarction, Hypertension, Diabetes and Obesity in Three Neighboring Communities in Pennsylvania. *Amer J. Med. Sci.* In press.

Chapter VII

THE MODIFICATION OF REACTION PATTERNS: THE THERAPEUTIC PROCESS

THE PATIENT PHYSICIAN RELATIONSHIP

IN THE INITIAL APPROACH to the patient an interested concern on the part of the physician is of utmost importance. When a patient feels secure that he is in the presence of a physician who is not only competent but sincerely interested in him, it becomes far easier to divulge pertinent information and provide the necessary data on which judgments are to be made. In this connection, the meticulously performed physical examination has considerable importance. Furthermore, the opportunity for the physician to appraise his patient, to search his own past experience, and to contemplate the immediate problem allows him to utilize what is popularly known as intuition (1-6).

In talking with the patient, the tacit communication that whatever he says or does, the patient is safe from censure, ridicule or betrayal, affords the best chance for a productive interview. Occasionally, remarkable "cures" may be effected through a single encounter with a physician that imparts to the patient a sense of dignity, of being respected, and of having a significant place in the scheme of things.

Patients have thus been rapidly freed from a paralysing sense of frustration, or the seemingly unbreakable shackles resulting from their own tortured but often unconscious conflicts (7). More often however, the process of "working through" personal problems to the abandonment of former costly patterns of adjustment, requires several interviews spaced sometimes close together or even separated by weeks or months (8). The development of a stable and satisfactory adjustment may require years of patient support and understanding by the physician. Such a relationship

229

often implies extreme and prolonged dependence of the patient on the physician. It may require extraordinary flexibility and sensitivity to cues on the part of the physician. He may be called upon to tolerate expressions of bitter hostility from his patient, broken appointments and wounds of pride. He may need to alter radically from time to time the frequency of visits, their duration and even his manner, vis a vis his patient. For the physician, such an approach to the patient's problem is costly in energy. It is not a method that can be used by those who can give but a few minutes to an interview. If, however, during the first few visits intensive and time-consuming studies of the patient's problems have been made, subsequent short visits may be adequate.

The physician should be aware of his own personal problems which might distort his judgment, provoke in him too much sympathy for the patient on the one hand, or on the other, arouse his irritability, antagonism, and feelings of disapproval. The physician's manner vis a vis the patient as mentioned above is of first importance. He should convey a warm personal interest and concern without features of familiarity. He must concern himself with the patient's problems, without becoming identified with them. Such skill in managing the interpersonal relationship of physician and patient lends immeasurably to the effectiveness of the physician (6).

The physician should aim to obtain facts, record them in chronological order and follow a plan, but yet not so rigidly as to impose it on the situation. He must utilize facts as they become available, especially to discover the attitudes and the reactions of the individual and then formulate the results of these studies and changes in behavior to the patient without cliches. He should avoid aimless or rambling dialogue and must not promise to eliminate the patient's obstacles or limitations. In fact the physician should appreciate that elimination of symptoms may demand more in personal adjustment than the patient is willing to give. It is the role of the physician to bring clearly into focus the cost to the patient of his manner of life.

The Interview

A rewarding initial approach is to have the patient relate in great detail the previous twenty-four-hour period of his life; then to outline the activities, feeling states, complaints and symptoms of the previous week; and to make a statement as to what he thinks may be related to his illness. It is well then to proceed further into the patient's past with a systematic and detailed survey of his biographic and personality features. If, however, the patient has had unusual and distressing experiences which he is anxious to tell about, it is best to allow him to do so immediately in order to release his tension. Also, the patient should immediately be urged to relate in detail the circumstances surrounding any exacerbation of symptoms that occurs during the period of interviews. Of more importance to the patient than awareness of immediate precipitating circumstance, is a broader understanding of the significant facets of his personality and life situation that persist and precede manifestations of illness by days or weeks. It is particularly helpful to correlate with care the exacerbations of symptoms with significant events in the patient's daily life and periods of particular vulnerability in the past. The recognition of such correlations may serve to convince the skeptical patient and engender his lively interest and cooperation, thereby greatly accelerating progress (see Fig. 1, p. 19). Certainly, for every patient his prompt and full appreciation of the truly poisonous and destructive nature of hate, resentment, jealousy, frustration, envy and fear is of crucial importance. In other words, the analysis and understanding of the genesis of pernicious attitudes and protective reaction patterns used inappropriately provide a kind of re-education. All such discussions should emphasize an alteration of attitudes and the development of a way of life within which the patient can pursue his day-to-day activities, with less and less costly emotional and bodily reactions.

The physician should watch for results in the patient's changed day-to-day performance rather than in changed verbalization. Even after a series of interviews when the daily performance and attitude of the patient have strikingly improved, he may still

make poor or totally inadequate verbalizations. A patient's formu-
lations are often quite different from his behavior, if for no
other reason than because of a limited facility in the use of words.
Also, persons change their behavior from time to time as situations
demand it of them, but since they are not called upon to formulate their experience and changing attitudes at the time, they
may in the future, when asked to state their position or attitude,
actually express a point of view that they have abandoned long
before.

The patient should be made to appreciate from the beginning
that there is no easy road to the goal he wishes to achieve, and
especially should he realize that sedatives and tranquilizers can
offer him no more than transient help.

Even though a destructive life situation exists and cannot be
improved, a patient's attitude may so markedly alter as to bring
acceptance, relaxation and a new capacity to cope with hitherto-
fore intolerable circumstances. A fixed unwillingness to change
may defeat all therapeutic effort.

Every interview with the patient assumes therapeutic possibilities as follows:

1. The patient sees in a detached way the nature of his
symptoms.

2. He realizes that his own problem must uitimately be
solved by himself in terms of his own equipment and experience;
the physician enables him to do this by directing attention to
this or that facet of his personality, emphasizing its potential
importance.

3. Through the physician's attitude of respect for situational
difficulties and the emotional reactions to them, the subject comes
to assign a new value to certain departments of his life which he
considered irrelevant or so intensely personal, as to have pre-
cluded review.

4. Almost every interview can terminate constructively, not
merely through reassurance or suggestion, but actually in terms
of some concept which the patient can fully appreciate and which
gives him new information as well as courage in dealing with
his problem.

5. There should usually be a concise and orderly formulation to the patient of the important facts that have been revealed and the relation of these to his complaints. By this means, the patient himself will often be able to see ways for correction. If he has failed to understand the formulation the next interview can begin with a restatement that he can grasp.

The physician should not be discouraged by the return of symptoms with mounting tension. Rediscussion of important points is sometimes necessary, since habits and attitudes often outlive the stress evoking life crises which gave rise to them. Insight does not always lead to new habits of behavior, and old habits are not easily broken. Sometimes, despite the best efforts at having the patient discover his own solutions, the physician will have to point to concrete means of adjustment.

Thus, it may be necessary actually to work out for the patient a new plan of life to which he should adhere closely. Such a plan should include details of occupation, recreation and rest.

A review of a patient's actual twenty-four-hour routine as mentioned above affords a convenient means of becoming familiar with the demands he makes upon himself and the standards to which he adheres. Direct questioning about stress seldom brings forth useful data, since many subjects are not aware of, or will not admit, states of tension, fatigue, weariness, boredom, or satiation with work. In order to discover the identity of stress-evoking circumstances it is essential to understand the personality of the subject, since a situation that would be of no significance to one individual may be highly charged for another. Or, further, circumstances that are easily weathered by a subject at one period of his life may produce evidences of stress at another. Thus, the subject must appreciate that ambitions and output of energy compatible with well-being at age twenty may not be so at age forty. In other words, demands that are compatible with comfort at twenty may produce difficulties at forty. Also, bodily symptoms often become manifest in subjects who fail to see themselves achieving the goals defined in their younger years and who have difficulty in altering their attitudes and their energy out-put. The patient may be mystified by his symptoms in the face of the fact that no dramatic deviation has occurred in the routine of his life. Since he cannot see the origin of his tension it is difficult for him to seek help.

The subject can be asked to list his self-appraised assets and contrast them with a similar list of his deficits. He then reveals not only his basic values but also he becomes aware of his own assets, assets he may have overlooked in his own self-appraisal.

Relief of anxiety and tension may be achieved through review with the subject of his list of self-appraised assets and deficits. Thus, he can often be encouraged to a better appreciation of himself. The physician may be able to engender confidence and security in the patient by dwelling on his assets and attempting to redirect his drives toward more satisfying goals.

Repeated review of the life story may help to reveal the dynamics of pernicious emotional states and explain feelings of guilt, inadequacy, and anger. The patient by becoming aware of the genesis of his moods and reactions may gradually or even promptly, become able first to accept and then to temper them.

Conventional psychological tests for aptitudes and intelligence and evaluation of actual performance may help to set more realistic goals.

THE RECOGNITION OF HAZARDS

Those who have had a strong need to repress and avoid facing their feelings and attitudes may be seriously endangered by the physician's approach which too quickly explores and uncovers unconscious material. Indeed, the unwary physician may suddenly find his patient utterly out of control, in an unmanageable panic, self accusatory and deeply depressed, suicidal or even disorganized in the manner of a schizophrenic. Such "last ditch" reaction patterns are evoked under extreme circumstances, as for example, when a patient discovers for the first time that he harbors murderous impulses toward his wife or other members of his family, or on his becoming aware of other attitudes within himself which his conscience would find unacceptable. Because of such hazards, many physicians must make a decision when or whether or not to refer a patient for psychiatric care. The decision is dependent on the physician's appraisal of his own capability and willingness to cope with the situation rather than on any rules of thumb or formal training experiences he may have had. In any case, referral for psychiatric care must be undertaken with adequate preparation and explanation to the patient and with no implication of abandonment. It is desirable to maintain continuity with the patient by some appropriate means.

EVALUATION OF PROGRESS

There is often striking improvement during the first few weeks of treatment because of the encouraging nature of the opportunity to talk freely without fear of censure, ridicule or betrayal, because of the infectious optimism of the physician, and because of other factors related to the novelty of the experience perhaps motivating the patient to perform well. Occasionally misleading to the physician is a patient's "flight into health" as a defense against further painful revelation of personal problems. Such spurious improvement may also be motivated by a desire to placate the physician. Even valid improvement rapidly achieved should not delude the physician into thinking that the patient's difficulties can be easily dispelled. Occasionally they can, with no need for further care, but more often the early period of remission is followed by discouraging exacerbations calling for continued effort by both patient and physician. Significant results of therapy will appear in subsequent months when the patient, hopefully with diminishing symptoms and increasing insight and energy, has had an opportunity to demonstrate his ability to establish a more satisfactory and long-lasting salutary pattern of behavior.

SOCIAL AGENCIES AND PARAMEDICAL PERSONNEL

More and more in modern medical practice the comprehensive and continuing care of the patient is provided not only by the physician but also by social service workers, public health nurses and a lengthening list of specialists whose efforts can be coordinated into a thorough going treatment plan. While a direct personal relationship with the physician is indispensable, help from these various agencies can spell the difference between therapeutic success and failure. The contribution of the social worker, sociologist, psychologist and certain other specialists may not only strengthen the therapeutic effort, but also provide important information for diagnosis and for establishing the goals and plan of therapy.

CHANGING ACTIVITIES

One of the most time-honored prescriptions for patients caught in stress evoking circumstances is a change of scene. Thus a vacation or even giving up one's urban job and moving to the country may be recommended.

The suggestion often made that a man may have to give up his work and change to a less exalted but more "healthful occupation" carries with it many hazards. "Mental life" so-called, is not necessarily the offending agent, but removal from an accustomed way of life with the introduction of more physical work and less "mental work" may solve the patient's problems. Even though transplanting sometimes achieves the end desired, it should be realized that it is not primarily the "exercise," "the fresh air," and contact with "the soil" that causes improvement, but the changes in attitudes and in pace, and the freedom from competition and tension. Unless the patient is able to accept and appreciate such advantages, the countryside may bring with it as many symptoms as the office or bank in the urban community.

Complete retirement from work is not usually a desirable therapeutic device, since work is often a major creative and social outlet. On the other hand, as mentioned above, work that is distasteful because of its incompatibility with the temperament and aims of the subject should be modified or abandoned.

The success of the change-of-scene prescription probably led to the widespread establishment of spas during the latter part of the last century. The spa with its atmosphere of being cared for, its tradition of healing, the freedom from decision through ordered menu, exercise, rest and social life, is helpful. So, also, is the long sea voyage. It is essential, however, that the therapeutic effectiveness of the spa or the sea voyage be attributed to the proper situational factors and not to certain chemical elements in the waters, or the freshness of the sea air. Sea bathing is also restorative to some individuals because of the relaxing effect of the sunlight, the diverting circumstances of the beach, and the relaxed air of gaiety common to seaside resorts.

Physical Therapy and Occupational Therapy

Exercise including games, massage and warm baths, cold baths, sun baths and heat treatments while lacking in specific qualities for the treatment of the symptoms associated with pernicious reaction patterns, nevertheless afford relaxation and release of tension for many and may promote better concentration, better sleep and restoration of energy. Frequently, a migraine headache can be aborted by a vigorous "work out" or a competitive game. Similarly, massage, hydrotherapy and heliotherapy may induce in some persons the desired state of relaxation. Many patients who gain very little from these measures may benefit from activities that are sufficiently interesting and challenging to divert them from troublesome preoccupations. Thus, hobbies and crafts and especially creative activity such as photography, writing, sculpture, painting, or playing the piano may afford a sense of accomplishment and satisfaction in addition to diversion. Most intelligent people are capable of creative activity of some sort but in our society few avail themselves of this rich source of satisfaction.

CHEMOTHERAPY

The most widely used chemotherapeutic agents are the barbitrates and "tranquilizers." Few of these agents have a specific effect on the disorders discussed in this volume although reserpine and some other agents in the tranquilizer group may reduce blood pressure. Reserpine, however, is a stimulant to gastric hydrochloric acid secretion and in large doses may aggravate or even precipitate a peptic ulcer. Another serious disadvantage of reserpine is its tendency to provoke depressive reactions, especially in hypertensive patients. Although barbiturates, and even "anti depressant agents" may be indicated to combat the patient's anguish, it is generally better to avoid their use and especially one should not attempt to substitute such agents for psychotherapy.

Certain pharmacodynamic agents are helpful in controlling the peripheral manifestations of the various diseases and disorders discussed such as a number of hypotensive agents, antacids and anticholinergic agents, analgesics, vasoconstrictor agents (i.e., ergotamine tartrate for vascular headache of the migraine type), bronchodilators and a host of other agents for specific symptoms.

Endocrine secretions involved in the homeostatic process also find application in therapy, especially epinephrine for asthma. The use of adrenocorticotrophic hormone and adrenocortical hormones has had an interesting history and has illuminated to some extent the pathogenic processes involved. They have been shown to aid in the restoration of homeostasis during shock after the abreactions to injury. Also, the stress phenomena exhibited as asthma, ulcerative colitis, and "fatigue" after excessive or sustained effort may be constructively modified. The reactions to non-specific noxious factors, shown as rheumatoid arthritis, the collagen syndromes, some varieties of chronic inflammation, and myasthenia gravis may be temporarily mitigated.

On the other hand, changes in the stomach and duodenum exhibiting themselves ultimately as peptic ulceration are worsened by corticosteroids as are dysfunctions of the cardiovascular system in which fluid and electrolyte balance are disturbed and in arterial hypertension. These agents may intensify epileptic phenomena or aggravate the metabolic manifestations of diabetes mellitus.

SURGERY

Complications and irreversible aspects of various of the reaction patterns may require correction by surgery, but the surgeon is rarely able to make a fundamental contribution to the elimination or effective alteration of reaction patterns. Thus, vagotomy for peptic ulcer, already referred to may bring periodic epigastric pain under control and may remove the hazards of hemorrhage, perforation and obstruction, but the procedure otherwise leaves the attitudes and reactions of the patient unchanged.

The distressing symptoms of the dumping syndrome, post prandial weakness, tachycardia, sweating and often nausea occur most often, according to surgical workers, when there has been a failure to reach a reasonable resolution of the patient's conflicts prior to operation. Indeed, most surgeons agree that the best operative results in peptic ulcer are observed in those patients who have acquired some understanding of the nature of their problems of adaptation.

Surgical measures directed at the highest integrative functions of the brain, the various frontal lobotomies, have found little application except in frankly psychotic individuals. The intellectual impoverishment which follows the destruction of a large number of cortical connections, while rarely incapacitating, is a sufficient handicap to preclude the use of the procedure in all except those who are overwhelmed by tension or obsessive preoccupations.

DISCUSSION

The therapeutic process calls for modification of disabling and potentially destructive reaction patterns. In addressing himself to this challenge, the physician must call on a vast array of medicaments and maneuvers, and in addition he must be aware of the fact that a fundamental alteration in a reaction pattern presupposes a change in the person's conscious and unconscious appraisal of his situation. The task of helping a patient achieve a truly realistic and fundamental reorientation requires the physician to assume responsibilities far greater than those of most of his recent predecessors and many of his contemporaries who have grown up in the age when attacks on bacterial agents of disease and disturbances in body chemistry have been so spectacularly successful. Today, as at times in the past, the man of medicine is called upon to understand the aspirations and the strivings of his patients and to afford assistance to them in divining a constructive purpose in life and in seeking an inner equilibrium. A century ago in this country such were the offices of the clergy. In recent years, a comparatively small sector of the population has turned to the clergy. Thus, a broader responsibility falls to the physician. While infections and physical forces that impinge on the patient continue to occupy the physician's attention, and while he must persist in attempting to mitigate their effects and relieve suffering, his major attention will need to be directed more and more against internal factors, and he should find himself functioning as a catalyst so that the sick one changes himself and external environmental factors operate less destructively.

To the uninitiated, it might appear impossible for a physician to help an adult patient make a fundamental alteration. Yet, man is amazingly plastic. He is continuously making new adjustments, new experiments with nature, sometimes adequately, often inadequately. The physician may be helpful as a figure of authority, one who affirms his belief in the individual, especially during tentative explorations in any new directions of adjustment. He becomes especially potent when he operates in an institution such as the hospital, symbolizing accumulated wisdom, tribal support and a tradition of compassion.

The keystone of such a process is the patient-physician relationship. Ultimately the question is whether, with such an orientation, the physician can effect a change in attitude and health. A significantly suggestive study of results of such efforts was made a few years ago at the New York Hospital in a special clinic (9, 10). Results achieved were appraised in terms of "constructive change" as regards: (1) the symptoms that brought the patient to the clinic; (2) other stress reactions ("signs and symptoms"), and (3) basic attitudes.

Seven hundred and thirty-nine persons were admitted to the New York Hospital experimental clinic with complaints or manifestations of stress of the various types that have been considered in the previous chapters of this monograph. These patients were described as regards improvement in symptoms noted during the three-year period of study. The average number of visits per person was about fifteen and the average number of hours of attendance per person was about nine. The data were as follows:

State	On Discharge 739	1 Yr. Later 367	2 Yrs. Later 196
No change	33.5%	29%	29%
Change in symptoms:			
Minor to moderate	42.5%	41%	43%
Major	24 %	30%	28%

The state of improvement remained approximately the same during the two or more years after a new adjustment had been made. Although there were differences as regards the degree of change, nonetheless, the summary grouping together in the way indicated did not do violence to the facts about individual syndromes (9, 10). Approximately two out of three persons were constructively altered. Thus, whereas minor to major constructive changes in the category of symptoms and other stress reactions occurred in about two-thirds, major alterations of basic attitudes were comparatively uncommon, occurring in only one-tenth to one-fifth of the group. Nevertheless, certain bodily changes themselves causing no symptoms, such as arterial hypertension, were altered to average levels for long periods when associated with a basic change in attitude. In patients in whom established and irreversible organic changes had occurred, major reversal of the bodily manifestations of stress were not achieved. Such were: pyloric occlusion from scarring; bleeding or perforation from peptic ulcer; fibrotic changes in the lung of an asthmatic; vascular changes in the kidneys of a hypertensive; mucosal and vascular damage with blood and fluid loss in ulcerative colitis. Yet, even in persons so gravely afflicted, the achievement of even a modest degree of tranquillity and freedom from sustained hostility and conflict were often strikingly associated with amelioration and sometimes disappearance of symptoms.

It is difficult to attribute improvement to a certain procedure without knowing what could have happened if another form of therapy had been offered. Accordingly, as a continuation of the Berle study, results achieved in patients with ulcerative colitis and peptic ulceration over a two-year period in the experimental clinic were compared with those achieved in matched patients in other medical clinics in the same period of time using conventional methods (12). The findings strongly favored the experimental clinic where the proportion of improved patients was twice that, and the mortality half that encountered in the conventional clinic. Furthermore, only a third as many patients in the experimental clinic underwent surgical intervention.

Thus, roughly two persons out of three with such stress manifestations as have been discussed can be relieved of their suffering and their ominous bodily reactions. Furthermore, about one in five can be so altered basically as to be relatively safe from recurrence.

BIBLIOGRAPHY

1. WOLF, S.: A new view of disease. *Trans. Amer. Clin. Climat. Ass., 74*:168-175, 1963. *J. Amer. Med. Ass., 184(2)*:129, 1963.
2. WOLFF, H. G.: *Headache and Other Head Pain.* New York, Oxford, 1948 and 1963.
3. BOGDONOFF, M. D., BREHM, L., and BOCK, K.: The effect of the experimenter's role upon the subject's response to an unpleasant task. *J. Psychosom, Res., 8*:137, 1964.
4. WOLF, S.: Asking the question. *Psychosom. Med., 24*:417, 1962.
5. WOLFF, H. G.: A concept of disease in man. *Psychosom. Med., 24*:25-30, 1962.
6. WOLF, S.: Talking with the patient. In: *Monographs in Medicine,* pp. 1. William B. Bean, Ed. Baltimore, Williams and Wilkins, 1952.
7. RIPLEY, HERBERT S., and WOLF, S.: The intravenous use of sodium amytal in psychosomatic disorders. *Psychosom. Med., 9(4)*:260-268, 1947.
8. WOLF, STEWART, and WOLFF, H. G.: *Headaches: Their Nature and Treatment.* Boston, Little, 1953.
9. BERLE, BEATRICE B., PINSKY, RUTH, WOLF, S., and WOLFF, H. G.: A clinical guide to prognosis in stress disease. *J.A.M.A., 149*: 1624, 1952.
10. RIPLEY, H. S., WOLF, S., and WOLFF, H. G.: Treatment in a psychosomatic clinic. Preliminary report, *J.A.M.A., 138*:949, 1948.
11. WOLFF, H. G., and WOLF, S., in collaboration with BERLE, B. B., RIPLEY, H. S., DUNN, W. H., and SHEPARD, E. M.: The management of hypertensive patients. In: *Hypertension, A Symposium.* E. T. Bell, Ed. Minneapolis, Univ. Minnesota Press, 1951.
12. GRACE, W. J., WOLF, S., and WOLFF, H. G.: *The Human Colon. An Experimental Study Based on Direct Observation of Four Fistulous Subjects.* New York, Hoeber, 1951.

Chapter VIII

FORMULATION

T HROUGHOUT THIS MONOGRAPH the highest integrative functions of the brain have been seen as responsible for the expression of human proclivities and for the fulfillment of human potentialities, as well as for numerous manifestations of disease. The thesis has been presented that the integrative function of the brain, dominant in the regulation and control of the viscera as well as the musculo-skeletal structures of the body, formulates patterns of adaptation to many stress-evoking circumstances which may be inappropriate in kind, amount and duration, and hence be ultimately disruptive, and even destructive. It appears, therefore, that a conspicuous portion of man's illnesses is a function of his goals, his methods of attaining them, and the conflicts they engender (1, 2).

In short, prolonged circumstances which are perceived as dangerous, as lonely, as hopeless, may drain a man of hope and of his health; but he is capable of enduring incredible burdens and taking cruel punishment when he has self-esteem, hope, purpose and belief in his fellows (3, 4, 5).

In anticipation of this revised edition of his book, Harold Wolff had planned to conclude with a brief summary of goal-directed behavior in man's adaptive reactions as they constitute the manifestations of health and disease. Since the task of organizing his thoughts into a faithful epitome is beyond their accomplishment, the editors have decided to conclude with a brief statement in the words of one of them. The essay that follows was written after years of close association with Harold Wolff, and contains much of his point of view. It was published prior to his death. He had read it several times and had expressed his agreement with the thesis presented.

DISEASE AS A WAY OF LIFE*
STEWART WOLF, M.D.

I. *Man and His Brain*

Presumably, the high development of the mammalian nervous system has been responsible for the continued presence of our class on the earth. The dinosaurs had far more formidable weapons of attack and defense than the mammals have, and yet they became extinct at about the time the mammalian design was developed in the course of evolution. Mammals are generally more vulnerable than reptiles, but they are also more adaptable. The integrative activity of their brains provides for maintaining the temperature of the blood more or less constant in the face of a variation of 100 degrees or more in the surrounding atmosphere. Also, mammals are able to adapt to wetness and dryness, to altitude, and to the wily predatory maneuvers of their enemies. It would appear, therefore, that the purpose of the brain may be not so much to maintain constancy of internal environment but rather to permit effective adaptations to changes in the external environment.

II. *The Nature of Disease*

The long controversy that raged a century ago about whether diseases were "entities" or fundamentally normal bodily functions gone wrong has no real meaning today. Physicians now consider most diseases to be distinct from one another insofar as they represent patterned responses or adaptations to noxious forces in the environment. They are thus both "normal" bodily functions in the sense that they are adaptive phenomena and "entities" to the degree that they are classifiable and separable, one from the other, on the basis of either causative factors or similarity of manifestations. Phenomena generally recognized as indications of disease include quantitative alterations in body temperature, arterial pressure, the formed elements of the blood, vasomotor

---

*Reproduced, slightly edited, from *Perspectives in Biology and Medicine*, presented as the Minot Lecture to the Section on Internal Medicine of the American Medical Association, Atlantic City, June 9, 1959.

activity and hemodynamic mechanisms, the secretory activity of glands, and certain biosynthetic functions like, for example, those which characterize the sequence of blood coagulation. Other manifestations of disease include vomiting, malaise, as well as headache and other pain; muscular weakness, alterations in mood and behavior, and loss of consciousness; alterations in amount and composition of blood, plasma, and excretory products; shifts in electrolyte concentration in various body compartments; immunological phenomena involving alterations in capillary permeability; excessive cell reproduction; and tissue changes such as hyperemia, edema, and necrosis. A great variety of diseases share these mechanisms and manifestations in different combinations. Many of these mechanisms, the manifestations of disease, have been shown to be subject to influence or control by the central nervous system acting through neural, vascular, or endocrine pathways (6-9).

Traditionally, physicians have been inclined to consider diseases more localized than they really are, often on the spurious assumption that they involve only a single organ or organ system. Thus, pneumonia is thought of as a disease of the lungs although many of its manifestations—including fever, leucocytosis, increased antibody titers, tachycardia, etc.—are brought about by changes in organs distant from the lungs, such as the brain, the bone marrow, the lymph nodes, and the heart. The widespread manifestations of disease are usually nicely patterned. In congestive heart failure, for example, delicately balanced chemical, circulatory, and renal adjustments are well known as well as several alterations in endocrine secretions, including antidiuretic hormone, aldosterone, thyroid hormone, and corticosteroids. Again, many of these mechanisms have been shown to be connected with the central nervous system.

Neural integration is a complex system involving receptor and effector activity and something connecting the two. The connection may be direct, as in a simple reflex arc, or roundabout through interposed fibers concerned with interpretation, association with learned experiences, and other neural impressions either on a conscious or unconscious level. Thus, neural integrative activity refers to what takes place between the delivery of an afferent impulse to the central nervous system and the formation of an efferent pattern of response. It may occur at several levels of the nervous system. When language or other types of symbolism are involved, the process must include the highest integrative level, the cerebral cortex. Thus, the ultimate effector pattern may often depend upon the peculiar meaning or significance of a circumstance or event to the particular individual concerned. MacLean has suggested that all afferent information may be available to the hippocampus, an area considered important to affective and visceral behavior (10).

Influx of afferent impulses does not necessarily imply sensation. The viscera provide a profusion of afferent impulses which are not felt but which can be recognized through action potentials picked up from various subcortical sites. Both Russian and American workers have picked up a feedback in the brain from simple movements of the stomach (11, 12). Such afferents may provide the stimulus for patterning adaptive reactions in disease. In fact, when the influence of the brain is removed, the general expressions of systemic diseases may be greatly altered. Philip Bard has shown that without the cerebral hemispheres but with the brain stem intact—including the hypothalamus— a cat will not react with fever to the injection of a pyrogenic substance (13). Anaphylactic reactions to powerful antigens have been blocked by anesthesia and, in animals, also by ablation of the tegmentum of the midbrain (14). Adaptations are accomplished through a rich complex of entero- as well as exteroceptor pathways that subserve interactions or transactions between various levels of the central nervous system and other bodily structures, especially the glands of internal secretion. Thus, neural activity may alter thyroid function (15), for example and, in turn, variations in the amount of thyroid hormone secreted may have a profound and long-lasting effect on oxygen uptake by the brain (16).

It has become customary to substitute the terms "input" and "output" for the classical designations "stimulus" and "response." Input information reaches the highest integrative levels of the nervous system by a variety of routes including the nerves and the blood. The signals may be electrical, mechanical, or chemical, each affecting a specialized type of receptor. If the resulting neural impulse reaches consciousness, it becomes a sensation. Whether or not sensory information reaches consciousness, however, does not necessarily determine the nature or extent of the reaction, or output, except as will, desire, or motivation may add to the picture. Moreover, emotional responses may be aroused, such as fear, anxiety, or resentment, with or without awareness of the original input. Also, with or without awareness, and with or without an emotion or feeling-state, responses may be formulated in terms of striving, creating, destroying, avoiding, and so forth. Thus, frustration of aims and misfortunes may as well lead (and perhaps be essential) to the growth and strengthening of a person as to maladaptive reactions. The degree to which energy fed into the organism through afferent channels is essential to his well-being has not as yet been established. Certain it is, however, that a challenge to adapt can promote welfare and productivity. Hans Vaihinger stated, "Man owes his mental development more to his enemies (adversities) than to his friends" (17). The oyster produces the pearl in response to a stress stimulus.

III. *Neural Activity and Disease Patterns*

English-speaking neurophysiologists for the most part do not formulate their findings in psychological terms despite the fact that they may be concerned with excitation and inhibition at the cortical level. As W. Grey Walter has put it, "Facts accumulate at a far higher rate than does the understanding of them" (18). As the facts relating the functions of the brain to those of the rest of the body have accumulated, they have had relatively little effect on the thinking of most psychiatrists, who continue to use such abstractions as "psychic energy" and "motivational force." Neither have the findings of the neurophysiologists been incorporated into the thinking of most clinical investigators whose special fields embrace the organs in question, such as the cardiovascular system, the lungs, the kidneys, and so forth. The languages of the neurophysiologist, the psychiatrist, and the clinical investigator in this country are so disparate as to make it very difficult for them to understand one another.

The Russians have not suffered this handicap, and, in fact, are a good deal further along than we are in understanding the relation of the nervous system to disease, thanks to the influence of a contemporary of William Osler named Botkin. He evolved a clinical theory based on the work of his compatriot Sechenov and called it "nervism." He proposed that most, if not all, bodily processes are subject to some sort of regulation by cortical mechanisms—or, in our terms, neural integrative activity. Sechenov, who had worked under Claude Bernard, was impressed not so much by the constancy of the "milieu interieur" as by its capacity to adapt, presumably under nervous control, to changes in the "milieu exterieur," and thus protect the organism. He expressed his ideas in a book called Reflexes of the Brain (19), which aroused severe criticism from orthodox official Czarist Russia and became identified with the growth of the philosophy of dialectical materialism and the resultant political changes. In the scientific world, it inspired Pavolov's experimental work and his discovery of the conditioned reflex. Since the death of Pavlov, his pupil Bykov, with a great number of collaborators, accumulated an enormous body of evidence relating afferent and efferent connections of the cerebral cortex to a wide variety of visceral functions, including tissue metabolism (6).

Convincing evidence of the power of the nervous system over the rest of the body may be adduced from our everyday experience and without the artifacts of laboratory experimentation. Such is the case when the stimulus is a symbol which has no intrinsic force of its own but which undergoes interpretation by the brain and thereby gains its power. Hearing words which impart good news or bad, seeing a frightening sight, smelling a reminiscent odor, or taking into the mouth a substance with a disgusting taste may provide appropriate input for a variety of complex effector activities in the body. Nausea, with accompanying changes in motor activity of the stomach and duodenum, can be produced not only by emetic drugs and vestibular stimulation, but, in a female patient, by a discussion of pregnancy (20). It has been shown that nausea is always accompanied by interruption of gastric motor activity, loss of gastric tonus, and usually a transitory increase in the contractile state of the duodenum. In this experiment, the mention of pregnancy was followed by a sudden cessation of vigorous waves of gastric motor activity, a transitory increase in the contractile state of the duodenum, and nausea. This condition might be called hyperemesis gravidarum praecox, because the young woman was not pregnant at the time. The mere discussion of the pregnancy made her ill. In a hospitalized soldier during the New Guinea campaign in World War II, it was possible to observe, fluoroscopically, complete cessation of gastric movements with accompanying nausea simply by initiating a discussion of lurking Japanese or the horrors of the jungle (21).

Studies with hypnosis have provided another source of data concerning the effects of the highest neural centers on bodily processes as described in detail on page 108. They indicate that neural integrative activity may determine, in part, the degree of tissue damage from trauma. Other evidence that innervation may be implicated in tissue reactivity was adduced by Coburn (22) in the case of rheumatic nodules and by Smith and associates (23) with respect to the experimental production of atrophic gastritis. Flavell has shown that the mechanisms responsible for hypertrophic pulmonary osteoarthropathy depend upon afferent impulses from the lung which is affected by the cancer or other primary lesions (24). More recently, Calvert and Brody have adduced evidence that the hepatic damage from carbon tetrachloride is dependent in part on the sympathetic innervation of the liver (25), and the studies of Hampton and associates indicate that the vagus is implicated in the process of fibrin synthesis (26). These preliminary but highly provocative observations on the importance of peripheral nerves to various tissue reactions are reinforced by the experiments of Eccles in which the peripheral nerves to the soleus and gastrocnemius were sectioned in the newborn kitten and resutured in reverse. After regeneration Eccles and Buller recorded slow muscle potential from the gastrocnemius (normally fast), and fast waves from the soleus (normally slow) (27).

Just as neural mechanisms are capable of setting in motion many of the manifestations of disease, so are they capable of mitigating them. The evidence lies in the often efficacious effects of placebo therapy and in the success of a physician in whom the patient has confidence. This idea was expressed well by Burton in *Anatomy of Melancholy.* "An empirick oft times and a silly chirurgeon doth more strange cures than a rational physician . . . because the patient puts his confidence in him . . . He doth the best cures, according to Hippocrates, in whom most trust" (28). William Osler recognized this when he said, "It is much more important to know what sort of a patient has a disease than what sort of a disease a patient has" (29).

A great deal of data concerning connections between the viscera and the highest integrative neural centers may be obtained from studies with placebos, which have been used for centuries by physicians who, under pressure to "do something," wish to do no harm. Traditionally, the function of the placebo was to pacify without actually benefiting the patient. The benefit, however, often proves to be unexpectedly lavish. Not only does the hopeful reassurance of placebos engender in patients a feeling of increased well-being, but recent experimental evidence has shown that placebo administration may be followed by substantial and measurable changes in bodily mechanisms. The objective data are available in published reports and include alterations in pulmonary, gastrointestinal, urogenital, and adrenocortical functions, among others (30). Therefore, since placebos do a great deal more than placate or pacify, a new definition may be offered as follows: A placebo effect is any effect attributable to a pill, potion, or procedure but not to its pharmacodynamic or specific properties. Placebo effects derive from the significance to the patient of the whole situation surrounding the therapeutic effort. A connection is thus implied between the particular end organ and the interpretive areas of the brain. Placebo effects may be mediated by autonomic pathways, by other neural channels, or through humoral mechanisms. Relatively few of the routes are really well understood, but it has been shown that virtually all organs and organ systems are capable of responding to stimuli arising out of meaningful situations.

The degree to which disturbances in the environment provoke disease patterns by activating neural structures is incompletely understood. Certainly the various specialized receptors such as baroreceptors, osmoreceptors, and chemoreceptors in blood vessels and in the brain itself are sensitive to minor changes in the composition of the blood, especially to reductions in oxygen tension or alterations in blood pH. In many instances, it is known that the efferent impulses activated thereby may result in widespread and often disabling bodily changes (31). Stimulation by electrodes implanted in the nervous system has produced disturbances in blood coagulation (32), renal function (33), and a variety of endocrine effects including hypertrophy of the thyroid (34). Manning, Hall, and Banting induced myocardial fibrosis in cats and dogs by prolonged stimulation of the vagus (35). Gunn and Friedman have shown that lesions in the aorta and coronary arteries of rabbits produced by atherogenic diets can be greatly accentuated by stimulating chronically implanted diencephalic electrodes (36). Lipemia was also significantly greater in the stimulated animals. Seifter and associates have attributed a lipid-mobilizing effect to the pituitary under neural control (37). In our own studies, elevations of serum lipids have been achieved in humans during emotionally charged experiences while they were on a rigidly controlled diet on a metabolic ward (38).

The processes of renal excretion provide an excellent example of the integrative activity of the central nervous system. Several of the mechanisms which govern the amount and concentration of urine excreted have been shown to be subject to the influence of neural impulses. The evidence in animals is derived from experiments in which parts of the nervous system are stimulated or ablated. In humans, the studies of Schottstaedt and his collaborators are particularly notable (39). They were able to observe a diuresis of sodium and water in healthy subjects on a constant fluid and electrolyte intake under circumstances in which aggressive feelings were aroused. On the other hand, a pronounced retention of both sodium and water occurred in their subjects under circumstances marked by dejection or restraint. The findings were confirmed and found to be of particular significance in a study of patients with borderline congestive heart failure (40).

Other examples have been found in the experimental studies on the nose (41), bladder (42), esophagus (43), colon (44), heart (45), and skin (46).

IV. *Stress*

Stress, for the purpose of this discussion, is present when the adaptive mechanisms of the living organism—in this instance, man—are taxed or strained. The widespread acceptance in medicine of the term "stress" has led to the assumption that stress is something specific from which one might anticipate a specific bodily response. On the contrary, a stress is about as specific as an experience and, through the integrative activity of the brain, may yield almost any kind of response—from invention or creation to surrender or death.

Important discoveries, works of art, and advances in thought have been made under circumstances of stress. Reaction to stress may thus be measured in terms of achievement, or of the development of fresh potentials—but also in terms of the maintenance of equilibrium or in terms of failure of adaptation, behavior disturbances, and disease. The variety of adaptations is legion and, therefore, the mechanisms subserving them must be similarly numerous. Selye, whose pioneer work brought into focus the concept of stress, emphasized the role of the pituitary-adrenal axis in the adaptive reactions of animals (47). How frequently the adrenal may be involved in intact man is still an unsettled question. Certainly, adrenocortical hormones do not produce all so-called stress reactions. Only a relatively stereotyped pattern of metabolic changes can be induced by the administration of adrenal steroids. Stressful experiences, on the other hand, may induce a great variety of changes, usually bidirectional and not necessarily typical of adrenocortical effect. For example, the stomach may oversecrete or stop secreting altogether, depending on the circumstances. There may be a diuresis or a retention of salt and water. Surely the adrenal could not directly produce all the alterations. Adrenal cortical secretion does, however, seem to be important to support such changes, and the central nervous system seems to be essential to give them their pattern (48).

V. *The Individual and His Disease*

The characteristics of an individual are partly inborn and partly acquired. Stimuli which are encountered in the course of

day-to-day living—situations which challenge, threaten, or satisfy
—may evoke characteristic patterns of reaction in each individual.
The stimulus does not necessarily determine the pattern of response. The determinants include genetic equipment and other
characteristics of the individual which may be acquired. Thus,
the effect of the stimulus must depend heavily on the prevailing
state of the organism. The pertinence of the stimulus as a de-
terminant of the pattern of response derives simply from the
fact that it is the most recent event. Neither can one explain
the phenomena observed in response to a symbolic stimulus in
terms of the degree of emotional vulnerability of a particular
subject or in terms of nervous imbalance. As obtains with respect
to exposure to infectious agents, it can simply be said that some
people adapt more smoothly and effectively than others and thus
remain healthier.

The proposition that bodily illness may stem more or less
directly from neural processes concerned with the formulation
and fulfillment of purposes seems appropriate enough and yet
difficult to accept fully. The dilemma in the minds of students of
disease has been expressed in confused terminology: in the term
"psychogenic," for example, and in the meaningless distinction
between "organic" and "functional." All diseases are at once
functional and organic in the sense that their expression is a
disturbance in function of some organ of the body with or without
associated structural change or tissue damage. Thus, the distinction between physical disease and mental disease has little
meaning since the brain is an integral part of the human organism.

Lest there be any misunderstanding, I should like to emphasize that there is no implication that disease processes are "psychogenic" in the sense that their cause may be traced to a
psychological conflict of some sort. The implication is rather that
the disease may be an aspect of an individual's "way of life." Here,
genetic influences must be of the first order of importance—and
indeed, we are learning rapidly of more and more disorders that
have major genetic determinants. On the other hand, the attitudes and emotional life of the patient may in part determine
penetrance. The individual's psychological "set" seems related
in some way to the pattern of organ functioning which constitutes

the bodily disturbance or disease. Nevertheless, attempts to delineate a personality profile characteristic for the various disease states thought to be related to emotional stress have not been fruitful. Neither have efforts at isolating a characteristic or "nuclear" emotional conflict. The best data relating to specificity has come from a study of attitudes (49, 50). An "attitude" is interpreted broadly as the way an individual interprets his position vis-a-vis a certain situation. Most people have a characteristic Weltanschauung, or way of looking at life; perhaps more precisely, a way of reacting when cornered or seriously threatened. The gambler takes a risk; the cautious person becomes more cautious; the fighter fights; and the fleer flees. As pointed out earlier the patient with migraine meets challenging circumstances by doing things longer than, harder than, and better than his neighbor (51). The alcoholic meets challenges by disengaging himself from responsibility. There are a multitude of such patterns. When they are highly developed within us, as was indecisiveness in Hamlet, and when they are indiscriminately used, they may contain the seeds of our ultimate destruction (52). Difficulty may arise when the pattern is strained, that is, when too much is demanded of it; or frustrated, as when some circumstance blocks its use; or altogether inappropriate to the solution of the problem at hand.

VI. *Reactions in Anticipation*

The biological meaning of reaction patterns and the often vexatious neural connections which subserve them may lie in the protective and adaptive development of the nervous system which allows the organism to act in anticipation of a stimulus or event. Dubos, in his important book Mirage of Health, called attention to this characteristic in the neural tissue in such lowly forms as sea urchins (53):

> Because light seems to be somewhat injurious to it, the sea urchin naturally tends to remain in dark places. Yet it responds to a sudden shadow falling upon its body by pointing its spine in the direction from which the shadow comes. This response is defensive, serving to protect the sea urchin from enemies that might have caused the shadow in approaching.

The reaction is elicited by the shadow, but it refers to some-thing symbolized by the shadow as is well known. Similar symbolic reactions reach a complex development in higher animals. In man indeed, practically all responses to things seen or heard are merely reactions to representative stimuli. Just as comparative studies in metabolism have revealed a remarkable unity in all the biochemical phenomena of life, so studies of behavior have brought out certain patterns which, formally at least, are common to all living beings.

Rushmer has observed characteristic changes in left ventricu-lar function in dogs accustomed to treadmill studies merely by showing the animal the treadmill switch (8). In man, a great variety of reactions in anticipation have been studied experi-mentally. Salivation or the flow of gastric juice in anticipation of eating are familiar examples.

A. DISTORTION OF THE ANTICIPATORY REACTION

It is common knowledge, and easily understood, that a man running a race has tachycardia and increased cardiac output with lowered peripheral resistance so that more blood is de-livered to his muscles. Precisely the same bodily reaction occurs in the man who is driving his automobile and suddenly hears the shrill whirr of a motorcycle policeman's siren. He is not running or even planning to run, if he is wise, and yet his cardiovascular apparatus behaves as if he were running, and as if his muscles needed added nourishment. Such a bodily re-action, "as if," implies that the mechanisms in question are connected with and capable of reacting to impulses from the highest integrative centers. Strong evidence in support of this inference is available in the study of Rushmer, who produced the hemodynamic changes of exercise through electrical stimu-lation of the brain without the animal's engaging in any move-ment whatever (8). The biological reaction "as if" occurs most typically in anticipation of some experience—the flow of saliva prior to the mouthing of a tasty morsel or the flow of acid gastric juice in the stomach of a hungry man. It is now equally well recognized that such bodily reactions, "as if," may occur when there is no conscious or obvious connection with the action to which the bodily changes are appropriate. The gastric juice may flow profusely when an individual is frustrated and hostile and quite without appetite. Present-day evidence indicates that such changes may be great in degree, long lasting, and involve processes which may operate as disease mechanisms, even ending in death (52).

B. THEORIES RELATING "AS IF" TO DISEASE

Essential hypertension: as if blood loss were threatened.— The only uniformly observable bodily change which characterizes essential hypertension is an increase in peripheral vascular resistance. It derives presumably from sustained arteriolar constriction. The biological purpose of such a reaction, when imposed upon an initially normal blood pressure, is difficult to perceive. When blood pressure is low, however, as in the shock from blood loss, the pressor response of increased peripheral resistance bolsters what would otherwise be a lagging blood flow throughout the body, and especially in the important areas of the brain and heart. Indeed, hypertension has been induced when cerebral blood flow has been reduced by a variety of means (54), and years ago Cohnheim proposed that essential hypertension developed as part of an effort of the body to better perfuse the brain (55). It has been found possible to induce experimentally and predictably an increase in peripheral resistance with an actual elevation of blood pressure during bloodletting from transfusion donors (45). Indeed, a blood pressure rise attributable to increased peripheral resistance was often encountered prior to the venapuncture and in anticipation of the blood loss. The striking similarity between the hemodynamic adaptive response to bloodletting and the disordered state of essential hypertension may be a matter of coincidence. On the other hand, the hypertensive patient might be viewed as overcompensating for an unconsciously anticipated injury or blood loss. Those who have studied hypertensive patients psychologically have found them poised for aggression but yet restraining any aggressive activity and avoiding conflict. An extremely ingenious experimental situation calculated to arouse and yet

restrain aggressive impulses was contrived by the Russian workers at the primate laboratory in Zukhumi (56). Baboons which
had become self-selected mates were separated. The female was
placed in a large cage with a strange male while her mate was
placed in a smaller cage alongside. The cuckolded male regularly
developed a sustained hypertension. It would be difficult to en-
vision a situation better suited to testing the effects of restrained
aggression.

   Duodenal ulcer: readiness to devour.—Apart from the lesion
in the duodenal mucosa, the only bodily change which is known
uniformly to accompany peptic ulcer disease is an excessive production of gastric hydrochloric acid and pepsin; excessive because
it is sustained rather than intermittent. Each of us at mealtime
secretes large amounts of gastric juices with a high concentration
of acid and pepsin appropriate to digestion. The gastric behavior
of a peptic ulcer patient is as if he were always devouring or
receiving nourishment. One of the most effective elements in the
treatment of the disease is more or less continuous feeding. In
the jungle period of Man's evolutionary development the appropriate thing to do with an opponent or adversay was to kill
and eat him. Thus the linking of gastric hypersecretion of acid
and pepsin with circumstances that aroused hostility or resentment may have been a purposeful pattern acquired through
mutation. Perhaps the pattern has not been obsolete long enough
for civilized man to have lost it through further mutations. It
has been observed and repeatedly confirmed that stressful circumstances in the lives of patients with peptic ulcer, especially
those that arouse hostile feelings, may be associated with
acceleration of the secretion of gastric acid and pepsin. It may
be more than coincidence, therefore, that those who have studied
patients with peptic ulcers from a psychological standpoint have
found them a lean, hungry, competitive lot.

   Diabetes mellitus: as if one were starving.—The characteristic
metabolic change in diabetes mellitus is a tendency to substitute
fat for glucose as fuel for metabolic needs. The circumstance
under such a response that would be most appropriate is starvation; and indeed, during starvation glucose breakdown is reserved
for the nervous tissues and the testes, the only obligatory burners

of glucose. The liver makes available the metabolites of fat as a source of energy for the remainder of the body (57). For years psychiatrists have pointed out the frequent association of obesity with diabetes and the psychological identification in the minds of diabetic patients of food with love. Juvenile diabetes is most commonly preceded by a period of obesity, and usually there is evidence of deprivation of love during the infantile period (58-60).

Coronary artery disease: effort as a way of life, the "Sisyphus" reaction.—The evidence whereby coronary artery disease is related to an increased serum concentration of cholesterol and lipids is still incomplete. Available data relating lipid mobilization to exercise, however, would indicate that in view of the relatively small amount of glucose available in the body, vigorous muscular activity inevitably requires the mobilization of lipids to satisfy energy needs. The patient with hyperlipemia behaves biologically as if he were undertaking or about to undertake vigorous effort. In the light of this, it is striking that four groups of investigators who have reported psychological studies of patients with coronary artery disease find them to be distinctly effort-oriented (61-64). In our own studies, we found these patients to have a strong desire to do things on their own. They felt a great need to be responsible for what they did and delegated authority with difficulty. Moreover, they showed very little tendency to rest between labors; instead of savoring the satisfactions of accomplishment, they went on to meet the next challenge. This suggested designating theirs the "Sisyphus" pattern since Sisyphus, when confined in Hades, was required to push a great rock up a steep hill; whenever he was near the top, the rock rolled down again and required that he continue this effort.

VII. *The Ecology of Health and Disease*

Since the days of Pasteur and until recently, medical thinkers have been preoccupied with the need to establish a single cause for disease processes. Such a concern has tended to obscure the evidence relating to the modulating power of the central nervous system on all sorts of noxious and potentially noxious experiences.

In fact, the weakness of the single-cause idea was recognized by some of the members of the French academy who had blocked Pasteur's appointment to that august body. One of his opponents, Pidoux, has said it as follows: "Disease is the common result of a variety of diverse external and internal causes (that) bring about the destruction of an organ by a number of roads which the hygienist and the physician must endeavor to close" (65). Thus, newer concepts of disease hold that illness and incapacity arise from efforts on the part of the body to deal with adverse forces in the environment more frequently than they do from the direct effect or intrinsic nature of the adverse stimulus itself. In a sense, disease is a reaction to rather than an effect of noxious forces. As each human organism may respond slightly differently, depending on genetic equipment, previous experience with disease, conditioning effects, and so forth, the manifestations of the same disease in different individuals will be variable.

Modern man is inclined to encounter noxious stimuli, or stresses of a symbolic nature, far more frequently than directly damaging assaults. His responses which, as we have seen, may involve his whole being in the direction of health or disease, depend upon his goals and values. Thus, they constitute his way of life. Throughout man's evolution, the quality of his performance has reflected the validity of his values. In terms of social as well as bodily health, he has often been more unadapted than adapted, more sick than well.

Among the adaptations required in modern Western civilization are many age-old ones and certain characteristically modern ones, including those inherent in a fluid social class structure. Other important factors are the conflict between Old World cultural pressures and those encountered in the United States as well as problems arising from instabilities in the family structure (52). The important fact that the body responds with disease patterns not only to tangible noxae, but just as readily to stimuli which owe their force not to their intrinsic qualities but to their meaning to the individual, forms the basis of the connection between the social sciences and medicine. Rudolph Virchow frequently insisted that medicine is a social science (66).

Cultural and social pressures share with universal psycho-

logical drives and inborn personal proclivities the ability to
shape or modify the interpretation of experience and thereby
bear upon the character of the bodily response that results.

Essentially, it appears that man needs to live in a fashion
acceptable to his fellows. He needs to derive spiritual nourishment from his activities and the things which happen to him,
and he needs to satisfy in some way his various emotional yearn-
ings, including his unquenchable thirst for power and prestige,
and to realize his potential for love and for creativity. Threats
to his ability to perform in all of these spheres constitute the important everyday stresses that are apparently behind so many
states of disability and disease. A preventive emphasis in medicine
demands that we take into consideration all of these factors and
that we attempt to develop satisfactory ways of dealing with them
individually and collectively.

We are gradually learning that in biology the only permanent
thing is change—change requiring new adaptive responses on
the part of organisms, races, and species to serve their need
to survive. Man's thinking brain has both aided him in his
adaptations and created new challenges for him. His science
and technology have provided protection from the elements and
from other destructive forces in the environment. At the same
time that they have endowed him with power beyond the wildest
dreams of the potentates of the past, they have also confronted
him with new hazards of injury, accidental death, and subtler
changes as well in the form of radiations and noxious chemicals
in the air he breaths and in the food he eats. Man's reckless
and apparently insatiable desire to explore and experiment has
led him to establish a kind of mastery over the world despite his
diminutive stature, the delicacy of his offspring, and his lack
of natural weapons such as sharp teeth or claws.

Disability and death resulting from exposure to the elements
were mitigated when man sought shelter and clothing; then the
wild predators were fended off with arms and the microbes with
public hygiene and antibiotics. Now, the illnesses related to
man's own productions and his relations with his fellow man
are gaining prominence. The creation of societies require that
males learn to live together without destroying each other; now
the survival of society requires that we learn to tolerate differences

in people and their points of view. The stress-fraught adaptations concerned with this step in development provide much of what is noxious in the environment of modern man. These forces combine with others that tradition has already acknowledged to limit him through disability and discomfort. It is with relevant and potentially relevant factors, then, that we must concern ourselves in examining disease mechanisms. Taking due cognizance of genetic proclivities, learned patterns of response, and pressures of all sorts—tangible and otherwise—we must look for the forces that arouse and the mechanisms that modulate adaptive efforts in the body.

EPITOME

It is fitting that the epitome of this presentation should be in the words of Harold Wolff from his essay. "The Mind-Body Relationship (1)."

"The unifying concept about man in relation to his environment put together on these pages is grounded on the recognition of the purposive, goal-directed activity inherent in living things, from the unfolding of a seed to man's pursuit of his highest aspirations. It is a concept in keeping with the facts of the goal-directed and self-regulating organization of all biologic systems, recognizing on the one hand the forces within the system that direct its development, form and functions, and on the other hand the molding influence of outside forces and changing relationships. It is a concept that requires that man be sensitive to the unfolding of his individual patterns, the kind of person he is, and the direction in which he can move. In a narrower sense, such a concept illuminates the nature of disease and gives it meaning; in a broader sense, it can serve as a basis for a philosophy. It is a concept that accounts for the destructive, inappropriate use of adaptive patterns when the individual perceives himself as threatened, not only where his own ends or self-survival are in question, but as well when spiritual or moral values are jeopardized. Sickness may ensue and his life may be dramatically shortened in his struggles for issues beyond himself. His aspirations and appetite for adventure may engender ominous conflict yet make possible growth to undefined limits."

BIBLIOGRAPHY

1. WOLFF, H. G.: *The Mind-Body Relationship.* An outline of man's knowledge. New York, Doubleday, 1960, Chap. 2, pp 43-72.
2. WOLFF, H. G.: Dormant human potential. *Arch. Neurol. (Chicago), 6*:261-263, 1962.
3. WOLFF, H. G.: Every man has his breaking point (?) The conduct of prisoners of war. *Milit. Med., 125*:85-104, 1960.
4. WOLFF, H. G.: What hope does for man. Science and Humanity Section, Saturday Review, pp 42-45, 1956 (Also reprinted and distributed by N. Y. State Committee on TB and P.H., and N. Y. State Heart Assn., Inc.) Also see: Has disease meaning? Soc. N. Y. Hosp. Rec., May 8, 1956, pp 10-17.
5. WOLF, S.: *Disease as a Way of Life: Neural Integration in Systemic Pathology.* Perspectives in Biol. and Med., Spring, 1960.
6. BYKOV, K. M.: *The Cerebral Cortex and the Internal Organs.* Trans. by W. Horsley Gantt. New York, Chem. Pub. Co., 1957.
7. SPERANSKY, U. D.: *A Basis for the Theory of Medicine.* New York, International Publishers, 1943.
8. RUSHMER, R. F., and SMITH, O. A.: Cardiac Control. *Physiol. Rev., 39*:41, 1959.
9. HOFF, E. C., and GREEN, H. D.: Cardiovascular reactions induced by electrical stimulation of the cerebral cortex. *Amer. J. Physiol., 117*:411, 1936.
10. MACLEAN, P. D., FLANIGAN, S., FLYNN, J. P., KIM, CHUL, and STEVENS, J. R.: Hippocampal function; tentative correlations of conditioning, EEG, drug and radioautographic studies. *Yale J. Biol. Med., 28*:380, 1955-56.
11. The central nervous system and human behavior. Russian Scientific Translation Program. Bethesda, National Institutes of Health, 1959.
12. DUNLOP, C. W.: Viscero-sensory and somato-sensory representation in the rhinencephalon. *Electroenceph. Clin. Neurophysiol., 10*:297, 1958.
13. BARD, P., and WOODS, J. W.: Central site of pyrogenic action of bacterial endotoxin. (Abst.) *The Physiologist.* Vols. 2-3, August, 1959.
14. FREEDMAN, D. X., and FENICHEL, G.: Effect of midbrain lesion on experimental allergy. *A.M.A. Arch. Neurol. & Psychiat., 79*:164, 1958.

15. HARRIS, G. W., and WOODS, J. W.: In: *Regulation and Mode of Action of Thyroid Hormones,* G. E. W. Wolstenholme and E. C. P. Millar, Eds. Boston, Little, 1957, p 3.

16. POTAPOVA, U. N.: Adrenalin and thyroxin in oxygen consumption in the sympathetic ganglia. *J. Physiol. (U.S.S.R.),* 25:805, 1938.

17. VAIHINGER, H.: *The Philosophy of "As If,"* Trans. by C. K. Ogden. London, Routledge, 1949, p 12.

18. WALTER, W. G.: *The Living Brain.* New York, Norton, 1953, p 275.

19. SECHENOV, I. M.: Selected works. Moscow, All Union Inst. of Experimental Medicine, 1935.

20. WOLF, S.: The evaluation of therapy in disease. *Trans. Amer. Clin. Climat. Ass.,* 66:61, 1954.

21. _____: Observations on the occurrence of nausea among combat soldiers. *Gastroenterology, 8*:15, 1947.

22. COBURN, A. F.: Some observations on the reactivity of the rheumatic subject. *Trans. Ass. Amer. Physicians, 73*:357, 1960.

23. SMITH, W. O., DUVAL, M. K., JOEL, W., HONSKA, W. L., and WOLF, S.: Further studies on experimentally induced atrophic gastritis in dogs. *Trans. Ass. Amer. Physicians, 73*:348, 1960.

24. FLAVELL, G.: Reversal of pulmonary hypertrophic osteoarthropathy by vagotomy. *Lancet, 1*:260, 1956.

25. CALVERT, D. N., and BRODY, T. M.: Role of the sympathetic nervous system in CCL_4 hepatotoxicity. *Amer. J. Physiol., 198*:669, 1960.

26. HAMPTON, J. W.: Neuro-regulatory mechanisms of blood clotting. Bull. 13, pg. 21, L. E. Phillips Psychobiological Div., Mt. Sinai Hosp. Research Center, Minneapolis, Minnesota, Feb., 1965.

27. BULLER, A. J., ECCLES, J. C., and ECCLES, R. M.: Interactions between motoneurones and muscles in respect to the characteristic speeds of their responses. *J. Physiol., 150*:417, 1960.

28. BURTON, R.: *Anatomy of Melancholy.* London, Chatto & Windus, 1891, p 168.

29. OSLER, W.: Quoted in: R. Dubos, *Mirage of Health,* New York, Harper, 1959, p 120.

30. WOLF, S.: The pharmacology of placebos. *Pharmacol. Rev., 11*: 689, 1959.

31. HEYMANS, C.: Reflexogenic areas of the cardiovascular system. *Perspect. Biol. Med., 3*:409, 1960.

32. GUNN, C. G., and HAMPTON, J. W.: CNS influence on plasma levels of factor VIII activity. *Amer. J. Physiol., 212*:124, 1967.

33. Hoff, E. C., Kell, J. F., Hastings, N., Shales, D. M., and Gray, E. H.: Vasomotor, cellular and functional changes produced in kidney by brain stimulation. *J. Neurophysiol., 14*:317, 1951.

34. D'Angelo, S. A.: Role of the hypothalamus in pituitary-thyroid interplay. *J. Endocr., 17*:286, 1958.

35. Manning, G. W., Hall, G. E., and Banting, F. G.: Vagus stimulation and the production of myocardial damage. *Canada. Med. Ass. J., 37*:314, 1937.

36. Gunn, C. G., Friedman, M., and Byers, S. O.: Effect of chronic hypothalamus stimulation upon cholesterol-induced atherosclerosis in the rabbit. *J.C.I., 39*:1963, 1960.

37. Seifter, J., Baeder, D., Zaraponetic, C., and Kalas, J.: In: *Hormones and Atherosclerosis*, G. Pincus, Ed. New York, Acad. Press, 1959.

38. Wolf, S., McCabe, W. R., Yamamoto, J., Adsett, C. A., and Schottstaedt, W. W.: Changes in serum lipids in relation to emotional stress during rigid control of diet and exercise. *Trans. Amer. Clin. and Climat. Assoc., 73*:162, 1961. Also: *Circulation, 26*:379, 1962.

39. Schottstaedt, W. W., Grace, W. J., and Wolff, H. G.: Life situations, behavior, attitudes, emotions and renal excretion of fluid and electrolytes: Retention of water and sodium. *J. Psychosom. Res., 1*:203, 1956.

40. Barnes, R., and Schottstaedt, W. W.: Relation of emotional state to renal excretion of fluid and electrolytes in patients with congestive heart failure. *Clin. Res., 6*:224, 1958 (abstract).

41. Holmes, R. H., Goodell, H., Wolf, S., and Wolff, H. G.: *The Nose*. Springfield, Thomas, 1950.

42. Straub, L. R., Ripley, H. S., and Wolf, S.: Disturbances of bladder function associated with emotional states. *J.A.M.A., 141*:1139, 1949.

43. Wolf, S., and Almy, T. P.: Experimental observations on cardiospasm in man. *Gastroenterology, 13*:401, 1949.

44. Grace, W. J., Wolf, S., and Wolff, H. G.: *The Human Colon*. New York, Hoeber, 1951.

45. Wolf, S., Cardon, P. S., Jr., Shepard, E. M., and Wolff, H. G.: *Life Stress and Essential Hypertension*. Baltimore, William & Wilkins, 1955.

46. Graham, D. T., and Wolf, S.: The pathogenesis of urticaria. Experimental study of life situations, emotions and cutaneous vascular reactions. *J.A.M.A., 143*:1396, 1950.

47. SELYE, H.: *The Physiology and Pathology of Exposure to Stress*. Montreal, Acta, Inc., 1950.

48. ENGEL, F. L., and FREDERICKS, J.: Contribution to the understanding of the mechanism of the permissive action of corticoids. *Proc. Soc. Exp. Biol. Med., 94*:593, 1957.

49. GRACE, W. J., and GRAHAM, D. T.: Relationship of specific attitudes and emotions to certain bodily diseases. *Psychosom., Med., 14*:243, 1952.

50. GRAHAM, D. T., STERN, J. A., and WINOKUR, G.: Experimental investigation of the specificity of attitude hypothesis in psychosomatic disease. *Psychosom. Med., 20*:446, 1958.

51. WOLFF, H. G.: *Headache and Other Pain*. New York, Oxford, 1948.

52. _____: *Stress and Disease*. Pub. No. 166, American lecture series. 1st Ed. Springfield, Thomas, 1953.

53. DUBOS, R.: *Mirage of Health*, p. 106.

54. GUYTON, A. M.: Acute hypertension in dogs with cerebral ischemia. *Amer. J. Physiol., 154*:45, 1948.

55. COHNHEIM, J. F.: *Lectures on General Pathology*. London, New Sydenham Society, 1890.

56. UTKIN, I. A.: *Theoretical and Practical Questions of Experimental Medicine and Biology in Monkeys*. New York, Pergamon Press 1960.

57. KEYS, A., BROZEK, J., HENSCHEL, A., MICHELSON, O., and TAYLOR, H. L.: In: *The Biology of Human Starvation*. Vol. I. Minneapolis, Univ. Minnesota Press, 1950.

58. HINKLE, L. E., JR., EVANS, F., and WOLF, S.: Studies in diabetes mellitus. III: Life history of three persons with labile diabetes, and relation of significant experiences in their lives to the onset and course of the disease. *Psychosom. Med., 13*:160, 1951.

59. DANIELS, G. E.: Present trends in the evaluation of psychic factors in diabetes mellitus. *Psychosom. Med., 1*:527, 1939.

60. DUNBAR, H. F.: *Emotions and Bodily Changes*. 2d ed. New York, Columbia Univ. Press, 1938.

61. GROOVER, M. E.: Clinical evaluation of a Public Health Program to prevent coronary artery disease. *Trans. Coll. Physicians Phila., 24*:105, 1957.

62. HAMMARSTEN, J. F., CATHEY, C. W., REDMONT, R., and WOLF, S.: Serum cholesterol, diet and stress in patients with coronary artery disease (abstract). *J. Clin. Invest., 36*:897, 1957 (abstract).

63. RUSSEK, J. E., and ZOHMAN, B.: Relative significance of heredity, diet and occupational stress in coronary heart disease of young adults. *Amer. J. Med. Sci., 235*:266, 1958.

64. FRIEDMAN, M., and ROSENMAN, R. H.: Association of specific overt behavior pattern with blood and cardiovascular findings. Blood cholesterol level, blood clotting time, incidence of arcus senilis and clinical coronary artery disease. *J.A.M.A., 169*:1286, 1959.

65. PIDOUX, H.: Quoted in: *Mirage of Health.*

66. VIRCHOW, R.: *Disease, Life and Man.* Stanford, Stanford Univ. Press, 1958.

INDEX

Axon reflex, 107, 108
  in relation to elaboration of
    neurokinin, 107

B

Baboon
  experimental hypertension in, 257
Back pain
  attitudes associated with, 140
Barbiturates, therapeutic application
  of, 273
Behavior, patterns of (*See also*
    Adaptive responses)
  displacement, 131-133
  effect of on functions of the brain,
    157
  fragmented, or incomplete, 143
  goal directed, 128
  "parsimony," 143
  purposive, 131
  schizophrenia-depersonalization,
    133
  significance of event in relation to,
    145-151
  stockbound, 135
  summative effects in, 142
Bernard, Claude, 176, 248
Black magic, 198
Bladder
  hyper- and hypofunction, 89-91
  integrative activity and, 251
Bleeding
  with tissue fragility, 58
Blindness, 42, 48
Blister formation, 109
Body temperature, 138, 186
Bone pointing, 179, 198
Bradycardia, 74, 87
Bradykinin, 40
Brain
  diencephalic stimulation and
    atherosclerosis, 251
  eating behavior and highest
    integrative levels, 95
  effects of stimulation of, 172
  historical review of knowledge of
    the brain, 165-176
  hypothalamus, 73
  loss of substance, 157

  neocortex, structure, 172
  patterns of adaptation and activity
    of the brain, 151-158
  relation to adaptive patterns, 73,
    82, 93
  relation to diabetic metabolism, 93
Brain damage
  acute anxiety states stimulating, 152
  failure of conditioning process with,
    182
  late sequellae of suffering and
    misery, 209
  relation to adaptation, 14
Brain function
  impairment of, by prolonged
    adversity, 157
  in relation to neurotic behavior,
    151-158
Brain wave response
  changes in, as part of adaptive
    reaction, 153
  decline of with repeated
    stimulation, 25
Breaking point
  categories of, 179-181
  concept of, 177
Breathing
  neural apparatus for control of, 174
Bronchi
  in stress disorders, 60-63
  role in adaptation, 49
Bronchiectasis, 63

C

Cancer
  and pulmonary osteoartheropathy,
    249
  epidemiology, 26
  in prison camps, 212
Cardiovascular function
  cardiac arrest, 72
  changes in heart rate with
    stimulation of the amygdala, 172
  coronary ischemia, 76
  glands regulating, 73
  hemodynamic mechanisms in
    hypertension, 78-83
  in the adaptive process, 251
  patterns in hypertension, 76

Cardiovascular function: (Cont.)
  stroke volume and cardiac
    output, 77
Catecholamines
  and emotional experience, 95
Cecum
  evagination of, 72
Cerebral blood flow, 256
Change, noxious nature of, 187-189,
    260
  and tuberculosis, 190-194
  disruptions of war, 191-192
  geographic dislocation, 197
  industrialization, 191
  rapid social change, 193, 197,
    200-208
Chemotherapeutic agents, 237-238
Chinese expatriates, 203-205
Cholesterol
  concentration associated with effort,
    83, 258
  in coronary heart disease, 84-88
Circadian cycle of adrenal function,
    151 (See also Cyclical behavior)
Class structure
  stratified society, 219
Cold hands
  in Raynaud's disease, 138
  related to significance of event, 147
Colitis (See Ulcerative colitis)
Colon
  in adaptive mechanisms, 251
  increased fragility of mucosa, 142
  patterns of disturbed motility, 71-72
Coma
  in ketosis, 92
Combat, reactions during, 180
Common cold, 61, 64
Concentration camp
  change in symptoms during,
    145-147
  depersonalization in, 133
Conditioning
  alpha blocking by auditory stimuli,
    152
  failure of, in acute anxiety states,
    152
  in disease mechanisms, 259

Constipation, 70-71
  associated attitudes, 139
Controls, 22, 24, 25
Coronary artery disease, 84-88 (See
    also Cardiovascular)
  characteristics of patients, 86, 258
Corticosteroids (See Hormones)
Coughing, 51, 62, 63
Cramps, abdominal, 72
Cranial vasculature
  amplitude of pulsations, 39-45
    measurement of, 15
  changes in sensitivity to histamine
    and norepinephrin in headache,
    44
  in migraine, 43-46
  in relation to headache, 40-48
  lability of, in headache, 43-46
Cyclical behavior, 149-151
  circadian cycle of adrenal function,
    151
  menstrual cycle, 151
  predictable cycle of psychotic
    behavior, 151
  variation in urine volume, 149

D

Dachryocystitis, 48
Darwin, Charles, 6
Dental caries, 66
Depression, 20
  associated with dieting, 95
  hazard in therapy, 234
  in organized adaptive reaction with
    excessive grief or hostility, 151
  in relation to salt and water
    retention, 89
  with colonic hypofunction, 73
  with gastric hypofunction, 70
Descartes, Rene (1596-1650 A.D.),
    167, 168
Diabetes Meliltus, 62
  attitudes in, 257-258
  characteristics of patients, 93
  intensified by steroid therapy, 238
  ketosis in, 146
  relation to pituitary secretion, 93
  relation to starvation, 92, 93, 257
  relation to stress, 92-93

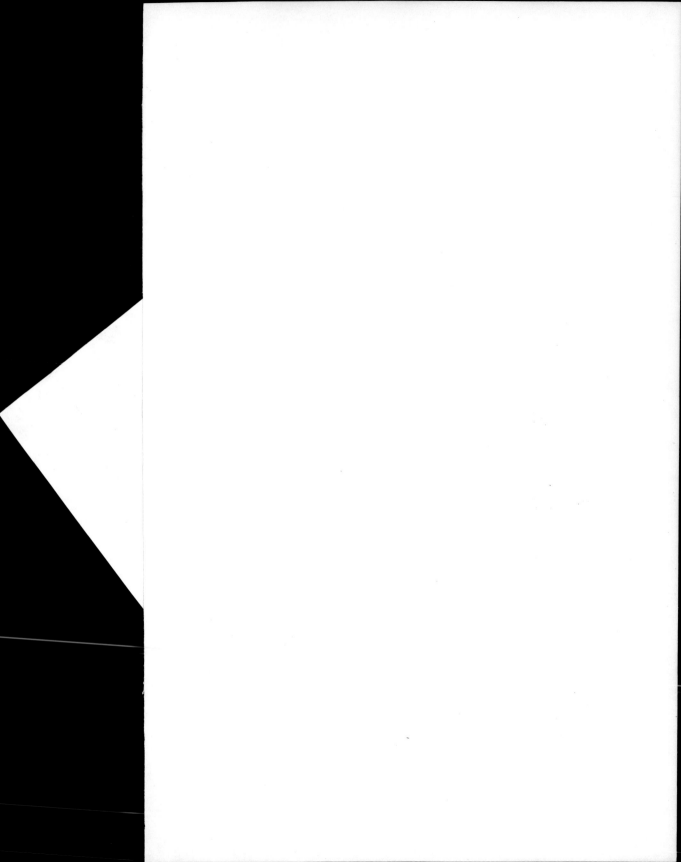

HOLY CROSS COLLEGE, NOTRE DAME, IN

DISCARDED

0 6000 000 268 494

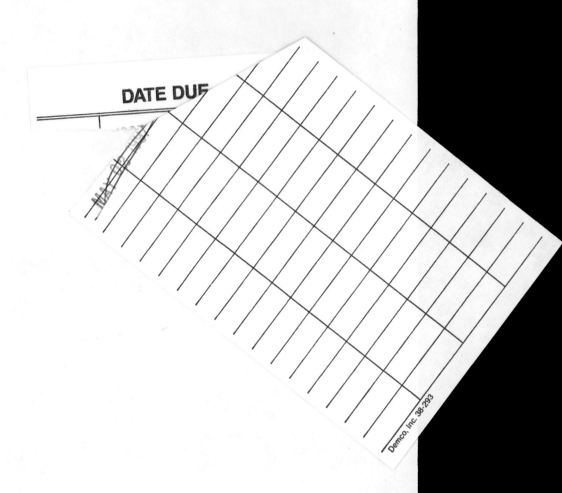

DATE DUE

Demco, Inc. 38-293